Sports and Exercise Training as Therapy in Cancer

Georg Stuebinger

Sports and Exercise Training as Therapy in Cancer

The Impact on the 24 Most Common and Deadliest Cancer Diseases Worldwide

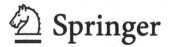

Georg Stuebinger
Graz, Austria

ISBN 978-3-658-14081-6   ISBN 978-3-658-09505-5 (eBook)
DOI 10.1007/978-3-658-09505-5

Springer
© Springer Fachmedien Wiesbaden 2015
Softcover reprint of the hardcover 1st edition 2015

Printed on acid-free paper

Springer is a brand of Springer Fachmedien Wiesbaden
Springer Fachmedien Wiesbaden is part of Springer Science+Business Media
(www.springer.com)

Foreword

I am a sport scientist and training therapist from Graz, Austria. This book covers the topic of a possible or well-established relation between sports and cancer. It gives an overview of what impact sports and exercise training may have or has got on each of the 24 most common and deadliest cancer diseases worldwide for all people interested or concerned with regard to the latest scientific findings. I am very engaged in this subject because of personal and occupational interests.

My heartfelt thanks to my whole family for your active support over the last few years and especially to my parents Mag. Christa Stuebinger und Klaus Stuebinger for your additional financial support to make it possible to release this book.

My master thesis, which was written at the university of Graz and advised by Univ.-Prof. Mag. Dr. Peter Hofmann, served as the general basis for this book.

Georg Stuebinger

Table of Contents

List of Tables

1 Introduction

Cancer is one of the major causes of death when all cancer types are pooled together accounting for approximately 13% of all deaths worldwide in 2008 according to the WHO while from 2008 - 2012, an increase from 12.677.000 - 14.090.149 new cancer cases resp. from 7.571.000 - 8.201.575 cancer deaths in more and less developed countries with higher percentages in incidence and mortality rates in 2012 in less developed countries.[1] [2] The following chapters are concerned with the impact of sports and exercise training at different types, durations, frequencies, volumes and intensities on prevention and reduced risk of cancer by means of every single of the 24 most common and deadliest types of cancer in men and women worldwide including proposed solutions and interesting questions for future studies.

Generally speaking, cancer represents a malignant tumor being increases or neoformations of several types of tissue like carcinomas in epithelial tissue or sarcomas in soft tissue whereby genes inside the nucleus of normal cells work in the wrong way by allowing a cell or cells to keep on dividing until a lump or tumor is formed, which can be benign that is not described as cancer due to traits of slow growth, a covering by normal cells, no spread into other body parts and cells being quite similar to normal cells, or malignant that is defined as cancer because of fast growth, the existence of cancer cells, the destruction of surrounding tissues, the entrance in blood vessels and the spread into other body parts.[3] To sum up, the main features of cancer are the resistance of cell death, the induction of angiogenesis, the enablement of replicative immortality, the activation of invasion and metastasis, the evasion of growth suppressors as well as the maintenance of proliferative signaling inclusive of deregulation of cellular energetics, avoid to be destructed by immune defense, tumor-promoting inflammation and genome instability and mutation.[4] During the emergence of cancer, proto-oncogenes become oncogenes controlling proteins being in turn responsible for ways of signal transduction after a mutation whereby the signal of growth is excessively increased due to overproduction of growth factors or receptors whereas simultaneously the impacts of tumor suppressor genes such as RB or p53 counteracting the effects of oncogenes and DNA repair genes are almost switched off.[4] p53 also inhibits glycolysis, but promotes aerobic metabolism and mitochondrial function resp. regulates the equilibrium of oxidative stress and antioxidative capacity being associated with reduced risk of cancer.[5] In cancer cells, the telomere representing a protective part of the DNA promoting cellular senescence (cellular aging) and apoptosis (cellular death) is also blocked by an enzyme called telomerase being able to add DNA being previously removed by telomere again as well as tumor angiogenic factors (TAFs) like vascular endothelial growth factor (VEGF) and transforming growth factor (TGF) are released to connect the cancer with neighbouring blood vessels so that the oxygen and nutrient demands can be ensured whereby metastases representing invasions into other tissues can arise because of the fact that those vessels, and also lymphatic vessels, are able to transport cancer cells being completely detached because cell adhesion molecules (CAMs) are missing in contrast to healthy cells.[4]

High-intensity sports and exercise training including an incremental endurance workout of continuous increases up to the maximal oxygen uptake (VO_{2max}) preceded by sufficient warm-up and recovery time increases the number of natural killer cells (NK) being able to kill cancer cells and also reduces the platelet-impeded cytotoxicity of NK-cells to cancer cells.[6] Cancer-induced cachexia representing progressive and significant weight loss accompanied by drastic catabolism of body fat and skeletal muscles affecting up to 50% of all cancer patients and being enhanced by pro-inflammatory cytokines promoting cell signaling such as tumor necrosis factor alpha (TNF-α) can also be warded off or relieved by pre-eminent resistance training due to the up-regulation of anti-inflammatory cytokines in body fat tissue and skeletal muscles by blocking TNF-α as well as increasing insulin sensitivity, muscle metabolism, protein synthesis and antioxidant enzymes.[7]

In comparison with the 70s, the 5-year relative survival rate for all cancer types significantly improved until today that can be elucidated by a combination of earlier detection and improved treatments.[8] [9] The increased incidence and decreased mortality rates of more or less developed countries are in turn mainly dependent on the cancer type, but not pre-eminently on the gender with the highest incidence rates and lowest mortality rates in more developed countries resp. the lowest incidence rates, but the highest mortality rates in less developed countries.[1] Referring to the metabolic situation in cancer cells, there is a much higher production of energy through glycolysis compared with healthy cells by converting glucose into lactate regardless whether the current level of oxygen is insufficient or not as well as without contribution of the oxidative phosphorylation in the mitochondria producing ATP as energy source, which is called the 'Warburg Effect' whereat a reverse 'Warburg Effect' was also recently discovered in tumor-associated fibroblasts being i. a. responsible for wound healing also resulting in a higher proliferative capacity by channeling the metabolites into the citric acid cycle. As a consequence, cancer cells as against healthy cells have got increased risk of tumorigenesis and carcinogenesis whereby an inhibition or a downshift of the glycolysis may be effective by opening new possibilities for immunotherapy on the account of a greater sensitivity of tumor and cancer cells.[10][11]

The main risk factors for cancer not listing all uninfluenceable risk factors such as inheritance account for smoking, alcohol use, low fruit and vegetable intake, obesity, contaminated injections in health care settings, unsafe sex, urban air pollution as well as physical inactivity.[12] Sports and exercise training seems to be a suitable adjuvant therapy for reduced risk of cancer because of the fact that on the one hand, sports and exercise training positively affects the hormonal and metabolic situation as well as inflammations, but on the other hand, also the risk of cardiovascular diseases and/or metabolic diseases possibly accompanying cancer due to weakened immune defense may be prevented or decreased by increasing physical fitness.[13][14] Moderate-to-high intensity sports and exercise training is considered to be an appropriate therapeutic agent in cancer prevention whereby the main focus has been on breast, prostate and colorectal cancer until now and every single type of cancer has to be differed from and considered incomparable to others whereas the role of sports and exercise training and its effects on tumor progression during and after chemotherapy still remains controversial whereby low-intensity sports and exercise training should not be ignored because of normalizing pH-value, decreasing lactate and inhibiting VEGF expression resulting in reduced angiogenesis in close vicinity to the cancer.[15][16]

All in all, sports and exercise training is safe and feasible for people to reduce the risk of cancer whereby physical and mental health benefits have been already proven as well as preventing obesity, cardiovascular resp. metabolic diseases whereas positive impacts of sports and exercise training on cancer progression and cancer survival may also be given.[17][18]

2 Sports & Exercise Training in Cancer

In the following chapter, the impact of sports and exercise training as a potential therapy on prevention and risk reduction of cancer is surveyed in detail as well as the palliative care for the 24 most common and deadliest cancer types in women and men worldwide. The order of cancer types was made by listing the cancer with the highest mortality rate of 2012 downwards to the cancer with the lowest mortality rate of 2012 worldwide.

2.1 Lung Cancer

Lung cancer represents the cancer with the highest mortality rate with 1.589.925 cancer deaths in 2012 worldwide by being the most common and deadliest cancer in 2012 among men resp. the 3rd most common and 2nd deadliest cancer in 2012 among women with an incidence rate of 1.241.601 new cases as well as a mortality rate of 1.098.702 deaths in 2012 among men resp. an incidence rate of 583.100 new cases as well as a mortality rate of 491.223 deaths in 2012 among women.[2] "The relative 5-year survival for patients with this disease is 14%, and has remained largely unchanged for years".[19] 85% - 90% are present as non-small cell lung cancers being subdivided into 25% - 30% of squamous cell carcinoma, 40% of adenocarcinoma and 10% - 15% of large cell carcinoma whereas 10% - 15% are present as small cell lung cancer.[20] Between 80% - 90% of lung cancer is attributable to smoking being unequivocally represented as the major risk factor, but risk factors appearing independently from smoking such as environmental tobacco smoke, cooking fumes, ionizing radiation, radon gas, asbestos, inherited genetic susceptibility, occupational exposures to carcinogens or pre-existing lung diseases accounting for ca. 10% - 15% of all lung cancers have also been confirmed as potential risk factors for lung cancer.[21] The risk of lung cancer in never-smokers is considered higher in women.[22] Important symptoms in patients with lung cancer are cough, dyspnea, hemoptysis, chest discomfort, phrenic nerve paralysis accompanied by bone pain, dysphagia, fever or clubbing.[23]

2.1.1 Sports & Exercise Training on Lung Cancer Incidence

A lack of physical activity can be associated with a higher risk owing to available data suggesting "moderate to high levels of leisure-time physical activity were associated with a 13% - 30% reduction in lung cancer".[24] A study accompanying 38.000 men from 1974 - 2003 ranging in age from 20 - 84 years and consisting of smokers and non-smokers evaluated a treadmill test. The people were assigned to low fit, moderately fit and high fit groups. The study illustrated that people with higher and moderate cardiorespiratory fitness levels may reduce the risk of getting lung cancer in comparison with those individuals with lower cardiorespiratory fitness levels.[25] The afore-noted outcome was also encouraged by a meta-analysis taking together the results of 7 different studies that also "indicate that moderate or high levels of leisure time physical activity are associated with reduced risk of developing lung cancer among smokers".[26] "Contrary to studies in smokers, ... data showed no evidence of inverse associations with higher BMI and increased physical activity" in never-smokers.[27] The correlation between physical activity and lung cancer risk in non-smokers in 230 cases and 648 controls was scrutinized in another study whereby physical activity of more than 24 MET-hours/week obtained the best results in never-smokers and ex-smokers.[28] 1 MET (metabolic equivalent) is the rate of energy expenditure at rest whereby intensities of physical activities under 3 METs are considered to be as light, between 3 and 6 METs as moderate resp. above 6 METs as vigorous. MET-hours are calculated by METs times minutes of physical activities divided by 60. The generation of reactive oxygen species (ROS) by oxidative stress working mutagenic can be well regulated by sports and exercise training to prevent oxidative damage and mechanisms of carcinogenesis transiently increasing ROS production, but in the long term, reducing the systemic ROS levels.[29] [30] Because of cancer cells producing energy by aerobic glycolysis resulting in high lactic acid levels, sports and exercise training combined with reduced carbohydrate availability contribute to increase the level of the tumor suppressor protein p53 that may benefit by a decrease of the glycolysis, a regulation of oxidative stress in the mitochondria as well as a protection against metabolic stress.[31] [32] Another study included 8 active male subjects performing a high-intensity endurance training with high or low carbohydrate availability whereby the maximal oxygen uptake (VO_{2max}) was settled at preliminary testing on the treadmill by 3-min. stages at 10, 12, 14 and 16 km/h and 2% inclination changes after the completion of 16 km/h until exhaustion. In the morning of the experimental trials being separated by a minimum of 7 days, the subjects performed a 50 min. bout of running on the treadmill being constituted of alternate 6 x 3 min. at 90% and 50% of the maximal oxygen uptake (VO_{2max}) whereat the warm-up and cool down lasted 7 min. at 70% of the VO_{2max} whereas the groups received CHO diets of 8g/kg (high) resp. 3g/kg (low) in the 24h before the experimental trials and a high-CHO breakfast comprising 2g/kg (high) as well as 8ml/kg resp. 3ml/kg of CHO beverages 10 min.

before and during recovery periods 2 and 5. Increases in p53 between pre- and post-exercise as well as between post-exercise and 3 hours after the interval training was shown while no increases were determined in the group with high CHO availability.[32]

2.1.2 Sports & Exercise Training on Lung Cancer Progression

The oxidative status of 16 lung cancer patients during a 14-week sports and exercise training period being comprised of 3 sessions per week was explored in a study and detected increases in urinary measures in postsurgical non-small cell lung cancer being able to promote cancer progression. "In week 1, exercise intensity was initially set at 60% of baseline peak workload for a duration of 15 to 20 minutes. Duration and/or intensity were then subsequently increased throughout weeks 2 to 4 up to 30 minutes at 65% peak workload. In weeks 5 and 6, exercise intensity varied between 60% - 65% of peak workload for a duration of 30 to 45 minutes for 2 sessions; in the remaining session patients cycled for 20 - 25 minutes at ventilatory threshold determined by a systematic increase in the VE/VO_2 ratio, while VE/VCO_2 remained constant. From the 7th week onwards, patients performed 2 sessions at 60% to 70% peak workload with one threshold workout for 20 - 30 minutes. Finally, in weeks 10 to 14, patients performed 2 sessions at 60% to 70% peak workload with one interval session. Interval workouts consisted of 30 sec. at peak workload followed by 60 s of active recovery for 10 - 15 intervals".[30] Higher levels of red cell distribution width (RDW) are also associated with advanced lung cancer stages, advanced age, more white blood cells, lower hemoglobin and higher levels of tumor markers.[33] Therefore 118 patients with chronic heart failure were supervised whereby the exercise group consisted of 71 patients resp. the control group of

47 patients. The exercise group completed a 6-month endurance training program of 3 weekly sessions of 60 min. each including an intensity of 90% of the heart rate at the anaerobic threshold (HR_{AT}), which was evaluated by cardiopulmonary testing on the treadmill being composed of a starting load of 20 or 40 W and incremental increases of 10 or 20 W every minute. The outcome indicates that high-intensity endurance training is associated with a decrease in RDW.[34]

2.1.3 Sports & Exercise Training on Lung Cancer Mortality

Relevant to the subject of performing sports and exercise training before lung cancer resection to improve pre-operative functional capacities and to decrease post-operative respiratory morbidity, 24 patients were randomly allocated into a group performing strength and endurance training (PR) and a group performing breathing exercises (CPT) for a period of 4 weeks and 20 sessions. The PR group performed a shoulder flexion with a minimum rate of 15 repetitions per min. resp. a treadmill run of 10 min. in week 1, 20 min. in week 2 and 30 min. in weeks 3 and 4 with the intensity of 80% of the maximum load that was determined by a test before and achieved better results compared to the CPT group performing 30 min. of inspiratory muscle training.[35]

2.1.4 Sports & Exercise Training on Palliative Care of Lung Cancer

Generally speaking, "exercise capacity is decreased due to lower peripheral muscle strength and pulmonary functions and increased dyspnea
severity and anxiety and depression levels in patients with advanced-
stage (stages III-IV) NSCLC and hence the quality of life of these patients is impaired much more in relation to reduced exercise capacity
compared to patients with early-stage (stages I-II) NSCLC".[36] Therefore,
articles of sports and exercise training prior to resp. post surgical resection were reviewed and occasioned results of endurance training lasting
30 or more min. per session performed three - five times per week at
moderate intensity of a 50% - 70% of the heart rate reserve (HR_{res}) being
calculated by maximal heart rate minus resting heart rate may have a
positive impact on sports and exercise training tolerance, the quality of
life and fatigue of early-stage lung cancer.[37]

2.2 Liver Cancer

Liver cancer represents the cancer with the 2nd highest mortality rate
with 745.533 cancer deaths in 2012 worldwide by being the 5th most
common and 2nd deadliest cancer in 2012 among men resp. the 9th most
common and 6th deadliest cancer in 2012 among women with an incidence rate of 554.369 new cases as well as a mortality rate of 521.041
deaths in 2012 among men resp. an incidence rate of 228.082 new cases
as well as a mortality rate of 224.492 deaths in 2012 among women.[2]
"The most common histological type of liver malignant neoplasm is
hepatocellular carcinoma (HCC). Other forms include: childhood
hepatoblastoma, and childhood cholangiocarcinoma (originating from

the intrahepatic biliary ducts) and angiosarcoma (from the intrahepatic blood vessels). The established risk factors for HCC include Hepatitis B or C viruses (HBV and HCV) infection, alcohol drinking, tobacco smoking, and aflatoxin. The suspected risk factors for liver cancer include diet, obesity, diabetes and insulin resistance, use of oral contraceptives, iron overload".[58] The major symptoms of liver cancer include drastic weight loss without any obvious explanation, swelling of the abdomen caused by growing cancer or a build up of fluid called ascites and jaundice as well as other symptoms like feeling full or bloated even after a small meal or loss of appetite over a few weeks or sudden health problems in people with chronic hepatitis or liver cirrhosis.[59]

2.2.1 Sports & Exercise Training on Liver Cancer Incidence

"Body mass index in both boys and girls during school age is positively associated with the risk of liver cancer in adulthood".[60] "In addition, diabetes mellitus, an important component of metabolic syndrome and risk factor for non-alcoholic fatty liver disease (NAFLD), has recently been associated with hepatocellular carcinoma (HCC) in patients with chronic liver diseases".[61] Physical activity levels of 6.093 participants at high risk of liver cancer were investigated by using accelerometers to measure frequency and intensity of regular physical activity (<100 counts/min./day = sedentary; 100 - 2.019 counts/min./day = light; 2.020 - 5.999 counts/min./day = moderate; > 6.000 counts/min./day = vigorous) with the final outcome that patients with a diagnosis of NAFLD, diabetes and metabolic syndrome have significantly reduced physical activity levels.[61] However, a resistance training of 3 weekly sessions of 60 min.

at 8 - 12 maximum repetitions each as well as consisting of 10 whole-
body exercises (leg press, leg extension, leg curl, chest press, lat pulldown, seated row, biceps curl, triceps extension, push-ups and sit-ups)
shows significant improvement in insulin sensitivity as compared with
an aerobic exercise of 3 weekly sessions of 40 min. at 50% of the maximal oxygen uptake at the point of voluntary stopping (VO_{2peak}) in week 1
and 60 min. at 60% - 75% of the maximal oxygen uptake at the point of
voluntary stopping (VO_{2peak}) by week 2 whereas health issues associated
with metabolic syndrome seem to be predominantly improved by endurance training of running about 12 miles or 120 min. per week at 65% -
80% of the maximal oxygen uptake at the point of voluntary stopping
(VO_{2peak}) as against resistance training of 3 weekly sessions of 3 daily
sets of 4 upper body and 4 lower body major muscle exercises of 8 - 12
maximum repetitions per set whereby performing the resistance training
in addition to the afore-noted endurance training brings along further
benefits.[62][63] Another study examined 19.921 NAFLD patients by performing an at least moderate-intensity sports and exercise training of 3,0
- 6,0 METs more than three times per week for at least 30 min. and for
an overall duration of at least 3 months, and reached the result that subjects who exercised regularly had a lower risk of having NAFLD and
were less insulin resistant.[64] 1 MET (metabolic equivalent) is the rate of
energy expenditure at rest whereby intensities of physical activities under 3 METs are considered to be as light, between 3 and 6 METs as
moderate resp. above 6 METs as vigorous. MET-hours are calculated by
METs times minutes of physical activities divided by 60. On the other
hand, short-term endurance training of 60 min. per session at 80% - 85%
of the maximal heart rate (HR_{max}) and performed for 7 consecutive days
also contribute to risk reduction of NAFLD and the following nonalcoholic steatohepatitis (NASH).[65] But "… whether NAFLD is a causative
factor for HCC remains unclear" although "NAFLD should be taken as a
risk factor for HCC".[66] Concerning a correlation between sports and

exercise training and hepatobiliary cancer also including liver cancer, a study contained 507.897 participants aged 50 - 71 by completing a baseline questionnaire of how often physical activity that increases respiration, heart rate or perspiration is done during a typical month whereby never (1), rarely (2), 1 to 3 times per month (3), 1 to 2 times per week (4), 3 to 4 times per week (5) and 5 or more times per week (6) were the options listed with the final result that the highest level of physical activity was significantly associated with a 36% risk reduction in total liver cancer as against physically inactive participants although in turn, HCC had a stronger association regarding reduction of liver cancer risk as compared with no significant associations in other liver cancer.[67] A number of studies "suggest that targeting insulin resistance and lipogenesis can reduce HCC risk over the long term" as well as "to prevent the onset of obesity through public awareness and education programs".[68] Considering the importance of cardiorespiratory fitness being associated with a lower risk of liver cancer, a treadmill test was performed in another study. The 38.801 male subjects aged 20 - 88 years were subsequently divided into low fit (lowest 20%), moderately fit (middle 40%) and high fit (upper 40%) groups and followed from 1974 until their date of death or December 31, 2003 with the final outcome that being a part of the moderately and high fit groups showed significant reduction of risk from liver cancer.[69]

2.2.2 Sports & Exercise Training on Liver Cancer Mortality

Sports and exercise training is considered to be an appropriate method for liver cancer patients undergoing hepatectomy. A study therefore allocates 51 HCC patients aged 20 - 80 years into a diet only and a combined diet and exercise group and testing their anaerobic thresholds one week after hepatectomy while the sports and exercise training program consisted of 3 resp. 5 - 6 weekly sessions of 60-min. walking and stretching sports and exercise training program and the diet program included a daily energy intake of 25 - 30 kcal/kg of body weight resp. 20 - 25 kcal/kg of BW in patients with diabetes or fatty livers, a daily protein intake of 1,0 - 1,2 g/kg of BW and a daily sodium chloride intake of 5 - 7 g/kg of BW, altogether during the 1-month preoperative and 6-month postoperative periods and came to the conclusion of a more obvious fat reduction and improvement in insulin resistance in patients of the combined group in comparison to the diet only group.[70] Another study carried out between December 2008 and April 2010, which included 61 HCC patients undergoing curative resection and being previously tested by cycle ergometry at 60 repetitions per minute (rpm) involving 2 min. incremental stages (5,0, 7,5 and 10W/min.) until the 60 rpm could not be pedaled any longer whereby the maximal oxygen uptake at the point of voluntary stopping (VO_{2peak}) as well as the anaerobic threshold (AT) was individually measured by breath-by-breath analysis of expired air. All patients were followed up at least every 3 months after discharge also inclusive of physical examination and liver function testing with the result that the 3-year survival rate in HCC patients with a level of the maximal oxygen uptake at the point of voluntary stopping (VO_{2peak}) of greater or equal 16,5 ml/min/kg was 50,3% as compared with 10,8% of those having less than 16,5 ml/min/kg and with an anaerobic threshold (AT) of greater or equal 11,5 ml/min/kg was 42,3% as against 33,4% of those having less than 11,5 ml/min/kg, but significantly higher 3-year survival rates were also achieved by higher platelet counts, branched-chain AA/tyrosine ratio (BTR) and albumin levels resp. lower aspartate transaminase (AST), alanine transaminase (ALT) and retinol-binding protein (RBP) levels.[71] A study found out that a 3-month treadmill-based

endurance training program being performed by 50 of 100 type-2 diabetes male patients aged 35 to 55 and consisting of 36 sessions altogether
of a 5 min. warm-up, a 30 min. main part at 65% - 75% of the maximal
heart rate (HR_{max}) and a 5 min. cool-down each significantly reduced
aspartate transaminase (AST) by 33,81% and alanine transaminase
(ALT) by 40,8% as against the control group.[72] Albumin synthesis is
significantly increased 5 hours after a 72-min. intensive and intermittent
endurance training at 85% of the maximal oxygen uptake at the point of
voluntary stopping (VO_{2peak}) in cycle ergometry while the ratio of aromatic to branched-chain AA may increase by endurance training in cycling conducted at a high-intensity of approximately 75% of the maximal
oxygen uptake (VO_{2max}) or even.[73 74]

2.2.3 Sports & Exercise Training on Palliative Care of Liver Cancer

Significant improvements in physical strength and endurance as well as
the quality of life was also determined by a study involving a 58-year-
old man with liver metastasis after resection of a carcinoma of the rec-
tum undergoing chemotherapy and consisting of a 13-week accompanying resistance training at 40% - 60% of the 1 repetition maximum and
endurance training at 130 - 150 heartbeats per minute (bpm) resp. at a
lactate level of 2 - 4 mmol/L for 10 min. each all being conducted twice
a week.[75] Moreover, another study examined a 55-year old male patient
suffering from advanced hepatocellular cancer (HCC) for 3 years from
then by letting him participate in a 6-week endurance training program in
cycling consisting of 2 weekly sessions of 20 min. in the first two and 35
min. in the last four weeks preceded by a 3- to 5-min. warm up and

followed by a 5 min. cool-down each. The intensity of the main part was 60% of the maximal heart rate (HR_{max}) that was priorly evaluated by an ergometric bicycle test also being performed after the 6 weeks and comprising a pedalling rate of 60 - 70 repetitions per minute (rpm) whereby the initial load of 20W was increased every 2 min. by 20W until exhaustion with the final result that physical working capacity and the quality of life were significantly up-regulated.[76]

2.3 Stomach Cancer

Stomach cancer represents the cancer with the 3rd highest mortality rate with 723.073 cancer deaths in 2012 worldwide by being the 4th most common and 3rd deadliest cancer in 2012 among men resp. the 5th most common and 5th deadliest cancer in 2012 among women with an incidence rate of 631.293 new cases as well as a mortality rate of 468.970 deaths in 2012 among men resp. an incidence rate of 320.301 new cases as well as a mortality rate of 254.103 deaths in 2012 among women.[2] Environmental and lifestyle factors associated with increased risk of stomach cancer include Helicobacter pylori being a microaerophilic bacterium in the stomach, smoking, salt, heavy alcohol consumption, high red meat consumption, high fat diets as well as low consumption of fruits, vegetables and micronutrients, obesity and physical inactivity.[94] But also "pre-existing diabetes mellitus may increase the risk of gastric cancer by approximately 19%" showing an either direct or indirect association between both diseases.[95] Symptoms of stomach resp. gastric cancer can range from abdominal pain, appetite loss, dysphagia, weight loss, vomiting in advanced stages to bloating, sudden early satiety, diarrhea, dyspepsia, shortness of breath and flatulence not being identified by stage whereby early stages are often asymptomatic.[96]

2.3.1 Sports & Exercise Training on Stomach Cancer Incidence

Referring to a correlation between sports and exercise training and stomach cancer risk, vigorous physical activity across periods of the lifespan may be inversely associated with stomach cancer risk whereby activity levels should be performed 3 or more times per week leading to approximately 20% - 40% risk reduction compared to the least active group whereas moderate sports and exercise training was not associated with reduced stomach cancer risk.[97] Another study involving 73.133 subjects being followed from 1984 - 2002 and interviewed by questionnaire to figure out individual sports and exercise training intensities, frequencies and durations in turn detected that durations between 31 and 60 min. at weekly frequencies of 1, 2 or more times as well as at primarily moderate intensity achieved the best outcomes whereby groups were differently full whereas BMI was not associated with risk of stomach cancer.[98] What this all amounts to is that a protective effect for stomach cancer may be given by certain higher levels of physical activity, although a protective impact is not entirely confirmed owing to a paucity of completed investigative studies.[99] Nevertheless "meta-analysis demonstrated that the risk of gastric cancer was 21% lower among the most physically active people as compared with the least physically active people ... . This protective effect was seen for gastric cancers in the cardia and distal stomach".[100] Generally speaking, people exercising 2 - 5 times per week including sessions lasting 30 or more min. each representing moderate-to high-intensity sports and exercise training levels significantly lower risk for stomach cancer.[101] Unfortunately, the actual intensities involving endurance and resistance training being required and useful to compile a sports and exercise training program are not available in current literature although an anaerobic threshold (AT) of less than 11 ml/min./kg and a concurrently low maximal oxygen uptake at the point of voluntary stopping (VO_{2peak}) also hint at higher rates of cardiopulmonary complications in patients with stomach cancer.[102]

2.3.2 Sports & Exercise Training on Stomach Cancer Progression

Regarding the natural killer cells being able to kill cancer cells, a study recruited 35 patients with stomach cancer aged 28 - 75 years having already undergone surgery and randomly allocated them into a control group doing no sports and exercise training as well as an exercise group carrying out a supervised 2-week sports and exercise training program comprising 3 daily sessions on 7 days per week lasting 30 min. of active range of motion (ROM) exercise, pelvic tilting exercise and isometric quadriceps-setting exercise each when patients lay in bed resp. consisting of 2 daily sessions on 5 days per week lasting 30 min. using arm and bicycle ergometers at moderate intensity each if patients were ambulatory with the final result that an early moderate sports and exercise training has got a beneficial effect on the function of NK cells in stomach cancer patients after surgery by significantly increasing the natural killer cell activity (NKCA) from 16,2% to 27,9% in the exercise group as compared with a decrease of natural killer cell activity (NKCA) from 19,7% to 13,3% in the control group.[103]

2.3.3 Sports & Exercise Training on Palliative Care of Stomach Cancer

Concerning a potential association of sports and exercise training in patients undergoing oral chemotherapy after surgery, 24 patients with stomach cancer were randomly assigned to a control group doing no sports and exercise training and an experimental group performing an 8-week home-based sports and exercise training program consisting of at least 3 weekly sessions of 20 - 30 min. walking at moderate intensity each preceded by a warm-up and followed by a cool-down including stretching of the upper and lower extremities as well as the hip joint with the final outcome that the ratio of natural killer cells being capable of killing off cancer and virus-infected cells was just as increased as the degree of the quality of life being evaluated by questionnaire just like decreases of cancer-related fatigue and anxiety.[104]

2.4 Colorectal Cancer

Colorectal cancer represents the cancer with the 4th highest mortality rate with 693.933 cancer deaths in 2012 worldwide by being the 3rd most common and 4th deadliest cancer in 2012 among men resp. the 2nd most common and 3rd deadliest cancer in 2012 among women with an incidence rate of 746.298 new cases as well as a mortality rate of 373.639 deaths in 2012 among men resp. an incidence rate of 614.304 new cases as well as a mortality rate of 320.294 deaths in 2012 among women.[2] Nonmodifiable risk factors include advanced age, adenomatous polyps, inflammatory bowel disease and inherited genetic risk whereas environmental risk factors include high-fat diets, high meat consumption, obesity, physical inactivity, cigarette smoking and heavy alcohol consumption.[77] "Exercise, whole-grain dietary fibre consumption and aspirin confer protection ... support the importance of environmental factors both in colorectal tumorigenesis and its possible prevention".[78] Some symptoms, especially weight loss and change in bowel habit, increase the risk of colorectal cancer when being accompanied by rectal bleeding being the predominant symptom, but conversely, other symptoms, such as decreased appetite, diarrhoe, constipation and perianal symptoms, seem to reduce the risk of colorectal cancer when being accompanied by rectal bleeding.[79]

2.4.1 Sports & Exercise Training on Colorectal Cancer Incidence

A study went through and reviewed a lot of studies and articles and ascertained that 75% of them showed either significant or non-significant reductions in risk of colorectal cancer with increasing physical activity.[80] Therefore, another study interviewed 488.720 men and women aged 50 - 71 years in 1995 and 1996 by baseline questionnaire about their intensities, frequencies and durations of performed sports and exercise training, and accompanied them until the end of 2003 and made out that among men and women, participants engaging themselves in sports and exercise training 5 or more times per week had the best outcomes and also had an 18% reduced risk of colorectal cancer as compared with those exercising never or rarely.[81] As a consequence, higher levels of physical activity serve as partly protective referring to the appearance of colorectal cancer although a protective association between levels of physical activity and colorectal cancer risk seems to be more consistent and stronger in men in comparison with women and more obvious for proximal colon cancer as against distal colon cancer and rectal cancer whereas the risk of rectal cancer alone was only reduced by a high level of vigorous physical activity.[82] [83] However, also "exercising one hour per week was associated with a lower prevalence of polyps and adenomas when compared to those who exercised less or not at all".[84] Generally speaking, sports and exercise training has got the potential of reducing the risk of colorectal cancer whereby the intensity has to be contemplated. Therefore, 952 rectal cancer cases being identified between May 1997 and January 2002 as well as 1.205 controls were recruited and interviewed by questionnaire about their intensities of physical activity and finally compared the results with 1.346 colon cancer cases being diagnosed between October 1991 and September 1994 as well as 1.544 controls aged 30 - 79 years each receiving the equal questionnaire as mentioned before. The final outcome indicated that the most reduction of colon and rectal cancer risk was determined by vigorous long-term activity levels of more than 12 hours per week in comparison with no reduction of colon cancer risk including all activity levels at moderate intensity and a minor reduction of rectal cancer risk inclusive of all activity levels at moderate intensity except between 2 - 5 hours per week at moderate intensity representing the significantly best result.[85]

2.4.2 Sports & Exercise Training on Colorectal Cancer Progression

In colorectal cancer, different kinds of chemokines, especially interleukin 8 (IL-8), belonging to the cytokines and inducing chemotaxis play a major role. Especially, expressions of growth-related oncogenes 2 and 3 (GRO-2 and GRO-3) are already increased in premalignant tumors as well as IL-8 levels are progressively increased in advanced colorectal cancer stages by 11-fold in adenomas, 30-fold or more in carcinomas and 47- to 80-fold in colorectal liver metastases indicating a significant association between IL-8 overexpression and progression and development of CRC by promoting tumor growth, metastasis, chemoresistance and angiogenesis that simultaneously implies that IL-8 being released by working muscles seems to be a suitable and notable therapeutic target in CRC, but higher levels of IL-8 based on a cutpoint of 2,41-fold of IL-8 overexpression counter-intuitively point towards a better overall survival rate.[86 87 88]

2.4.3 Sports & Exercise Training on Colorectal Cancer Mortality

On the other hand, "in multivariate analysis, women with a prediagnostic physical activity level of 18 or more MET-hours/week had a significantly lower colorectal cancer-specific mortality (32% reduction) and all-cause mortality (37% reduction) compared with women who reported no physical activity".[89] 1 MET (metabolic equivalent) is the rate of energy expenditure at rest whereby intensities of physical activities under 3 METs are considered to be as light, between 3 and 6 METs as moderate resp. above 6 METs as vigorous. MET-hours are calculated by METs times minutes of physical activities divided by 60. Concerning the afore-remarked counter-intuitive better survival rate, "exercise can increase plasma levels of various chemokines and cytokines, including IL-8 ... in healthy individuals" while a significant decrease of IL-8 levels is observed in patients with metabolic syndrome doing a 12-week moderate endurance training consisting of 3 weekly sessions of 40 - 50 min. of walking at 50% - 60% of the heart rate reserve (HR_{res}) being calculated by maximal heart rate minus resting heart rate.[90 91]

2.4.4 Sports & Exercise Training on Palliative Care of Colorectal Cancer

In relation to positive postsurgical impacts of sports and exercise training, a study recruited 31 stages I - III colon cancer patients aged 20 - 70 years between January 2011 and December 2011 for participation in a sports and exercise training program consisting of stretching for neck, shoulder, wrist, ankle and pelvis and very-low intensity resistance training of pelvic tilt, ankle dorsi- and plantar flexion against the hand of the therapist in phase 1 where patients were unable to get out of bed, of whole-body stretching and 10-sec. isometric resistance training involving pelvic tilt and thrust, leg raise, crunch, frontal and lateral raises and triceps extension in phase 2 where patients were able to get out of bed, but had limited ambulation as well as of whole-body stretching and phase 2 resistance training including 3 sets of 12 repetitions in addition to supervised balance exercises of one leg standing, one leg calf-raise, hip adduction, hip abduction, hip flexion with knee bent, hip extension and unsupervised walking on the hallway in phase 3 where patients were able to ambulate without any discomfort and figured out that low-to-moderate intensity sports and exercise training performed directly after colectomy reduces length of hospital stay by 1 or 2 days and improves bowel motility.[92] Though, also the mobility, fatigue and the quality of life in patients with stage IV colorectal cancer can be improved by a home-based sports and exercise training program embracing 5 upper body (biceps curl, rowing, pull down, bat swing, chest press) and 5 lower body (squats, calf raise, front, side and back steps) strength exercises performed at least twice a week for a total of 4 sessions (2 upper and 2 lower) at 10 - 15 repetitions with less than moderate exertion as well as endurance training of at least 4 weekly sessions of consisting of briswalking of about 1 mile per 20 min. lasting 90 min. each.[93]

2.5 Breast Cancer

Breast cancer represents the cancer with the 5th highest mortality rate with 521.907 cancer deaths in 2012 worldwide by being the most common and deadliest cancer in 2012 among women with an incidence rate of 1.676.633 new cases as well as a mortality rate of 521.907 deaths in 2012 among women.[2] But even so men can suffer from breast cancer although it is a rare disease and accounts for less than 1% of all types of cancer in males.[38] "The risk factors for breast cancer … include environmental factors such as radiation, tobacco, a high-fat diet, and xenoestrogens as well as hormones. In addition, BRCA1 and BRCA2 are the most well-known genetic factors that increase risk for breast cancer".[39] A study also revealed that the environmental risk factors for breast cancer are predominantly attributed to oxidative stress. Clear symptoms or apparent health problems for early diagnosis of breast cancer are lumps in the breast being either self-detected by women or determined by physicians.

2.5.1 Sports & Exercise Training on Breast Cancer Incidence

14.811 women aged 20 - 83 years were investigated by performing maximal treadmill exercise testing being finally allocated into a low (lowest 20%), a moderate (next 40%) and a high (upper 40%) group based on the individual performance capability and resulting in 33% and 55% lower breast cancer risk in women with moderate and high cardiorespiratory fitness levels.[40] "Physical activity may mediate breast cancer recurrence ... by reducing the levels of oestrogen in the body or by shifting the metabolism of oestrogen to favour production of 2-hydroxyestrone (2-OHE1) as opposed to 16alpha-hydroxyestrone (OHE1), the former of which has much weaker oestrogenic activity".[41] Relevant to the subject above, a total of 10 healthy, premenopausal and eumenorrheic women aged 25 - 35 years and classified at high risk of breast cancer, were recruited in a study lasting 7 menstrual cycles and consisting of a home-based sports and exercise training program on a treadmill altogether lasting 12 weeks and starting after the 2nd menstrual cycle whereby 3 women did not remain until completion of the study. Each participant had to perform 3 weekly sessions of overall 150 min. in weeks 1 and 2, 200 min. in weeks 3 and 4, 225 min. in weeks 5 and 6, 250 min. in weeks 7 and 8, 275 min. in weeks 10 and 11 as well as 300 min. in weeks 11 and 12 whereby one session had to last at least 15 min., but was not allowed to exceed 100 min. including an intensity of 80% - 85% of the maximal heart rate (HR_{max}) being primarily evaluated by an incremental treadmill test. The outcome provided evidence of lower total estrogen and total progesterone levels whereas the menstrual cycle length was not influenced.[42] Another study involved 79.124 women practicing walking and running between 1991 and 1993, 1998 and 2001 as well as 1999 and 2001 by questionnaires and got to the bottom of an increased breast cancer risk for women with larger cup sizes whereby estrogen and progesterone levels were the higher the larger the cup size. An interesting correlation between cup size and sports and exercise training extent was a significant decrease of estrogen and progesterone levels in women running or walking more than 25,0 MET-hours per week that may reduce the breast cancer risk and mortality.[43] 1 MET (metabolic equivalent) is the rate of energy expenditure at rest whereby intensities of physical activities under 3 METs are considered to be as light, between 3 and 6 METs as moderate resp. above 6 METs as vigorous. MET-hours are calculated by METs times minutes of physical activities divided by 60. The duration obviously plays a decisive role in endocrine symptoms when extending over a longer period of time and not coming equal or below 30 min.[44] [45] Other circulating sexual and growth hormones increasing the potential breast cancer risk, especially among premenopausal women, are estradiol, estrone, androstenedione, dehydroepiandrosterone and testosterone, but also postmenopausal breast cancer risk may be increased up to twofold in women with high estrogen or androgen levels.[46] [47] Another study reached the conclusion of decreased levels of estrone, estradiol, testosterone and androstenedione by doing combined reduced-calorie weight loss diet being comprised of a daily energy intake of 1.200 - 2.000 kcal including 30% or less from fat and moderate- to vigorous-intensity endurance training on the treadmill consisting of a 12-month sports and exercise training intervention of 5 weekly sessions of 225 min. per week at an intensity of 70% - 85% of the maximal heart rate (HR_{max}) measured by a maximal graded treadmill test by previously allocating 439 postmenopausal women aged 50 - 75 into 4 groups (control, only diet, only exercise, diet + exercise) and comparing the outcomes.[48] With the same duration and frequency as before, but a slightly modified intensity of 70% - 80% of the maximal heart rate (HR_{max}), 320 postmenopausal women were explored and significant reductions in estradiol were detected.[49] Another important topic to explore the impact of sports and exercise training is BRCA1/2 mutation carriers having a lifetime risk estimation for breast cancer of 30% - 80%. The results showed significant decreases in breast cancer risk for a medium level of 11,0 - 22,7 MET-hours per week inclusive of a medium level of intensity and a duration of more than 3,3 hours per week.[50] Another survey containing pre- and post-menopausal women irrespective of BRCA1/2 mutation carriers came to the result that post-menopausal women with a level above 22,9 MET-hours per week showed reduced breast cancer risk in comparison to pre-menopausal women at the same intensity as mentioned before not being associated with reduced breast cancer risk.[51] Generally speaking, endurance training seems to be a far more appropriate method when compared to 3 weekly 50 - 60 min. sessions of a 12-week resistance training involving 8 whole-body exercises (chest press, leg extension, shoulder press, leg curl, lat pulldown, leg press, biceps curl and triceps extension) of 2 - 4 sets per exercise at 8 - 12 maximum repetitions with 2 - 3 min. breaks between exercises and 30 sec. rests between sets because of the reason that significant increases in growth hormones including estrogen and testosterone were found in women that would be simultaneously counterproductive in the reduction of breast cancer risk and mortality rate.[52] "Considering intensity of sports and exercise training, stronger association was found between breast cancer risk and vigorous activity".[53]

2.5.2 Sports & Exercise Training on Breast Cancer Mortality

Standard recommendations for a supporting sports and exercise training against breast cancer cover an area of doing at least 20 to more advisable 60 min. of continuous endurance and resistance training regardless whether short bouts are incorporated, but including large muscle groups at an overall frequency of at least 3 – 5 times per week at an intensity of 50% - 75% of the maximal oxygen uptake at the point of voluntary stopping (VO_{2peak}), 60% - 80% of the maximal heart rate (HR_{max}) or a rate of perceived exertion (RPE) of 11 - 14 of a scale from 6 (very light) - 20 (very hard) to finally increase cardiorespiratory fitness levels of breast cancer patients being simultaneously coupled with an increased survival rate in the follow-up contemporaneously attended with energy balance control, well-balanced nutrition and sufficient fruit and vegetable consumption.[54][55] An interesting correlation between cup size and sports and exercise training extent was a decrease of estrogen and progesterone levels in women running or walking more than 25,0 MET-hours per week that may reduce the breast cancer risk and mortality.[48]

2.5.3 Sports & Exercise Training on Palliative Care of Breast Cancer

Sports and exercise training is often inversely associated with breast cancer risk and also "… improves the QOL and the overall physical fitness of breast cancer survivors following a brief (8-week) exercise program".[56] Regarding breast cancer patients undergoing chemotherapy, sports and exercise training seems to be an appropriate adjuvant method to increase or maintain physical capacity resp. to improve worsening symptoms whereby the intensity has to receive closer attention. A study assigned 301 breast cancer patients into a group performing 25 - 30 min. of endurance training (STAN), a group performing 50 - 60 min. of endurance training (HIGH) and a group performing 50 - 60 min. of combined endurance and resistance training (COMB) three times per week and merely during chemotherapy each with the final outcome that the HIGH- and COMB-groups achieved unambiguously better results in the management of declines in physical functioning and worsening symptoms. In detail, the HIGH-group was superior to the COMB-group for decreases in bodily pain and increases in physical fitness whereas the COMB-group was superior to the HIGH-group for improvements of muscular strength.[44] Endurance training is also seen as suitable to increase sports and exercise training tolerance and to decline dyspnea while receiving radiotherapy being determined by a study containing 46 female breast cancer patients performing a 6-week endurance training in cycling consisting of 5 weekly sessions of 40 min. cycling at an intensity of 65% - 70% of the maximal heart rate (HR_{max}) preceded by a 2 min. warm-up and followed by a 3 min. relaxation period and group breathing exercises. Endurance training was conducted 23 hours after receiving radiotherapy being composed of 7 weekly treatments for 5 weeks resp. sports and exercise training tolerance was determined by a 6-minute walking test including measurements of walked distance, dyspnea scale, blood pressure, heart rate and oxygen saturation.[57]

2.6 Esophageal Cancer

Esophageal cancer represents the cancer with the 6th highest mortality rate with 400.169 cancer deaths in 2012 worldwide by being the 8th most common and 7th deadliest cancer in 2012 among men resp. the 14th most common and 9th deadliest cancer in 2012 among women with an incidence rate of 323.008 new cases as well as a mortality rate of 281.217 deaths in 2012 among men resp. an incidence rate of 132.776 new cases as well as a mortality rate of 118.952 deaths in 2012 among women.[2] Esophageal cancer is subdivided into esophageal squamous cell carcinoma (ESCC) emanating from skin and mucosas, and esophageal adenocarcinoma (EA) springing from glandular tissue. Potential risk factors for ESCC include tobacco smoking, heavy alcohol consumption, drinking mate, low fruit and vegetable consumption, and achalasia whereas potential risk factors for EA contain gastroesophageal reflux, obesity, tobacco smoking, hiatal hernia, achalasia and probably absence of helicobacter pylori in the stomach.[116] "Often, esophageal cancer is not diagnosed until patients present with dysphagia, odynophagia, anemia or weight loss. When symptoms occur, the stage is often stage III or greater".[117]

2.6.1 Sports & Exercise Training on Esophageal Cancer Incidence

Increased sports and exercise training lasting 20 or more min. being performed a few times per week and causing increases in breathing, sweating and/or heart rate is positively associated with reduced risk of esophageal cancer, especially with EA, whereas no significant association is seen between sports or exercise training and ESCC.[118]An analysis including 8 studies attending to associations between sports and exercise training and reduced risk of esophageal cancer was conducted and finally arrived at the result that the risk of esophageal cancer was 19% lower among the most active people as against the least active people whereby physical activity was merely associated with a reduced risk of EA, but not of ESCC.[119] "Such mechanisms would include physical activity's affect on immune function, hormone levels, antioxidant defenses, overweight and gastroesophageal reflux".[120] The gastroesophageal reflux disease (GERD) or colloquially speaking heartburn or pyrosis arising from a chronic mucosal damage and being strongly associated with obesity can also represent a substantial risk factor for esophageal cancer as well as Barrett's esophagus being characterized as metaplasia and hence as a pre-malignant condition arising from GERD.[121] There is a possible association between insulin resistance and GERD symptoms and also the prevalence of erosive esophagitis whereby sports and exercise training combined with caloric restriction may be advantageous to decrease symptoms and complications of GERD as well as improve the quality of life in obese patients with GERD.[122] Because a dysfunction of the lower esophageal sphincter (LES) is a root cause of GERD, though it was also determined that LES pressure has got nothing to do with any level of physical activity although the LES pressure merely slightly declined in the group with the highest level of physical activity performing 8190 +/- 4320 MET-minutes per week.[123] But also after an esophagectomy, already low-level physical activity of 9 or more MET-hours per week seems to play a crucial role in preventing postoperative complications in comparison with other patients doing less or no sports and exercise training.[124] 1 MET (metabolic equivalent) is the rate of energy expenditure at rest whereby intensities of physical activities under 3 METs are considered to be as light, between 3 and 6 METs as moderate resp. above 6 METs as vigorous. MET-hours are calculated by METs times minutes of physical activities divided by 60.

2.7 Head and Neck Cancer

Head and neck cancer embraces four types of cancer including lip/oral cavity (39% in men resp. 58% in women), laryngeal (27% in men resp. 11% in women), nasopharangeal (12% in men resp. 15% in women) as well as other pharangeal (22% in men resp. 16% in women) cancers and altogether represents the cancer with the 7th highest mortality rate with

375.665 cancer deaths in 2012 worldwide by being the 6th most common and 6th deadliest cancer in 2012 among men resp. the 10th most common and 11th deadliest cancer in 2012 among women with an incidence rate of 513.104 new cases as well as a mortality rate of 284.555 deaths in 2012 among men resp. an incidence rate of 173.224 new cases as well as a mortality rate of 91.110 deaths in 2012 among women.[2] Head and Neck cancer predominantly appears as squamous cell carcinoma (SCCHN) whereby nearly 75% of all SCCHN attend to heavy tobacco and alcohol consumptions as primary causes, but also the Human Papillomavirus (HPV) may play a substantial role as a potential risk factor.[125] But also poor oral hygiene can play a role herein because "no regular dental visits and brushing teeth less than twice daily were associated with a significantly increased risk of head and neck cancer".[126] Anorexia, dysphagia or mouth sores can be early symptoms of head and neck cancer also being able to lead to reduced dietary intake and/or weight loss.[127]

2.7.1 Sports & Exercise Training on Head and Neck Cancer Incidence

To explore the association between sports and exercise training and head and neck cancer, a study recruited and interviewed 487.732 men and women without cancer aged 50 - 71 years from 1995 or 1996 to the end of 2003 by mailed questionnaire with the final outcome that people exercising 3 or 4 times per week had relative risks (RR) of total head and neck cancer and oral cavity cancer of 0,57 as against those exercising less than one time per week or nothing resp. that people exercising 5 or more times per week had relative risks of pharyngeal cancer of 0,48 and of laryngeal cancer of 0,52 as compared with those exercising less than one time per week or nothing.[128]

2.7.2 Sports & Exercise Training on Head and Neck Cancer Progression

A reason for beneficial effects of sports and exercise training in head and neck cancer are higher IL-6 levels in patients with head and neck cancer because of health behaviours, smoking or sleep disturbances among others whereby a 4 - 6 time per week performed endurance training including a running distance of 49 +/- 3 weekly km significantly decreases the level of IL-6 in older and younger people.[129][130]

2.7.3 Sports & Exercise Training on Palliative Care of Head and Neck Cancer

A study detected that functional capacity and the quality of life of patients undergoing chemoradiotherapy of head and neck cancer and participating in a 6-week sports and exercise training program consisting of 15 - 20 min. of brisk walking and of a resistance training program of the major muscles of the upper and lower limb including 8 - 10 repetitions and 2 - 3 sets each exercise at 3 - 5 of rate of perceived exertion (RPE) ranging from 1 - 10 and five times per week each was significantly improved as against a control group doing no sports and exercise training.[131] Another study conducted included 39 male and 10 female patients with stage III - IV of oral cavity, oropharyngeal, hypopharyngeal, nasopharyngeal or laryngeal cancers aged 32 - 78 years who underwent chemoradiotherapy and were randomly allocated into a standard rehabilitation group (S) performing a 10-week sports and exercise training program consisting of 3 weekly sessions of stretching the swallowing and jaw muscles by holding at mild discomfort for 10 - 30 sec. resp.

strengthening them by 8 - 12 repetitions per exercise and into an experimental rehabilitation group (E) by doing the same intensities and durations whereby a TheraBite was used to carry out exercises. The final result showed improvements with either of the two afore-stated sports and exercise training methods described above.[132] The mouthpieces of the TheraBite being predominantly used in trismus being well-known as a complication of head and neck cancer treatment must be positioned between the maxilla and the mandible whereby stretching is done when the handle of the TheraBite is squeezed and strengthening when the mouthpiece is squeezed. 69 head and neck cancer patients with trismus conducting sports and exercise training with the TheraBite from 2004 - 2011 involving 4 - 5 daily sessions of strengthening for 6 - 8 repetitions and stretching for 6 - 15 sec. were investigated with the final conclusion that mouth opening of head and neck cancer patients was increased by 5,4 mm after TheraBite exercises on average.[133] Resistance training also represents an appropriate method by increasing lean body mass and muscle strength in head and neck cancer for what another study recruited 41 patients with stage I and II head and neck cancers after radiotherapy and randomly assigned them into an exercise group performing a 12-week resistance training comprising 2 - 3 weekly sessions of 2 - 3 sets of 8 - 15 repetitions of 7 exercises including leg press, knee extension, hamstring curls, chest press, sit ups, back extensions as well as lateral pull down and into a control group performing no sports and exercise training.[134]

2.8 Pancreatic Cancer

Pancreatic Cancer represents the cancer with the 8th highest mortality rate with 330.391 cancer deaths in 2012 worldwide by being the 12th most common and 8th deadliest cancer in 2012 among men resp. the 12th most common and 7th deadliest cancer in 2012 among women with an incidence rate of 178.161 new cases as well as a mortality rate of 173.827 deaths in 2012 among men resp. an incidence rate of 159.711 new cases as well as a mortality rate of 156.564 deaths in 2012 among women.[2] The greatest risk factor for pancreatic cancer is chronic pancreatitis while acute pancreatitis, smoking, heavy alcohol consumption, long-standing diabetes, abnormal glucose tolerance, gallstones as well as autoimmune and infectious diseases play a major or minor role.[164][165] Epigastric abdominal pain getting worse when lying down, weight loss linked to less appetite, nausea with vomition after food intake, fat malabsorption and jaundice caused by a compression of the distal bile duct are the most common symptoms whereby an enlarged liver and a palpable gallbladder is present very often while anorexia, dyspepsia, pyrosis, depression, asthenia, thrombophlebitis, new-onset diabetes mellitus and gastrointestinal bleeding can also appear.[166] With the lowest survival rates among all cancer types, most patients suffering from pancreatic cancer succumb to the disease also because there is no simple early detection method and a resistance to chemotherapy.[167]

2.8.1 Sports & Exercise Training on Pancreatic Cancer Incidence

Concerning a possible correlation between sports and exercise training and pancreatic cancer risk, a study found 26 studies analyzing physical activity whereby the intensity of physical activity appeared more protective when being moderate as against vigorous or exhaustive whereat it is not significant and there is no state of evidence for potential effectiveness.[168] Diabetes mellitus is deemed to be a key factor for increased risk of pancreatic cancer, with a 1,5- to 2-fold elevated risk in type 2 DM whereas type 1 DM is associated with an increased risk to a lesser extent although the causality would be more apparent due to the fact that it is a dysfunction of the pancreas itself as against a mainly self-imposed insulin resistance representing type 2 DM whereby a clear state of evidence in both cases remains unclear despite of significantly increased risk for pancreatic cancer in older diabetic patients regardless whether type 1 or 2 diabetes lasting 2 years or less and/or comorbid with chronic pancreatitis.[169 170] Because of the fact, that there is no other way of dealing with type 1 DM as regular injections of insulin, sports and exercise training can merely help to reduce additional cardiovascular risk factors, improve metabolic control and lower HbA1c levels by 150 or more min. of intensive sports and exercise training whereat it has to be individually adjusted like type 2 DM as well to prevent adverse effects such as diabetic coma or hypoglycemia, but cannot avoid or cure type 1 DM.[171 172] HbA1c is a value being increased in type 1 and 2 DM and representing hemoglobin bound to glucose without enzymes. It can also be lowered by a 16-week combined 5 - 20 min. eccentric resistance training of the major leg muscles on a recumbent stepper at 7 - 13 on the rate of perceived exertion (RPE) scale ranging from 6 - 20 and 20 - 50 min. endurance training at 60% of the maximal heart rate (HR_{max}) on the treadmill, rowing machine, bicycle or elliptical stepper comprising 3 weekly sessions in type 2 DM patients whereby combined endurance and resistance training of 3 weekly 60 min. sessions involving 20 min. of cycling at 60% of the maximal oxygen uptake at the point of voluntary stopping (VO_{2peak}) and whole-body exercises (bench press, shoulder press, biceps curls, triceps extensions, sit-ups and leg press) of 1 set of 10 - 15 maximum repetitions improves the lipid profile of type 2 DM patients including reduced fasting blood glucose, HBA1c, total cholesterol, LDL-cholesterol, triglycerides as well as increased HDL-cholesterol, but resistance training seems to have more advantages in increasing insulin sensitivity and changes in lipid profiles.[173][174][175] The most potential risk factor for pancreatic cancer, pancreatitis, cannot be cured or prevented by sports and exercise training as well whereas possible risk factors for pancreatitis such as hyperlipidemia or gallstones can be prevented. On the other hand, high-intensity sports and exercise training could also induce pancreatitis as well as cholangitis after biliary bypasses or pancreatoduodenectomy.[176]

2.9 Prostate Cancer

Prostate cancer represents the cancer with the 9th highest mortality rate with 307.481 cancer deaths in 2012 worldwide by being the 2nd most common and 5th deadliest cancer in 2012 among men with an incidence rate of 1.111.689 new cases as well as a mortality rate of 307.481 deaths in 2012 among men.[2] "Recent smoking history, taller height, higher BMI, family history, and high intakes of total energy, calcium and α-linolenic acid were associated with a statistically significant increased risk. Higher vigorous physical activity level was associated with lower risk".[146] Symptoms of prostate cancer are lower urinary tract symptoms (LUTS) including hesitancy, leakage, urgency, dysuria, weak stream, frequency or alguria whereby early prostate cancer in stages I and II doesn't or rarely cause LUTS, but advanced prostate cancer in stages III and IV may or do cause LUTS.[147]

2.9.1 Sports & Exercise Training on Prostate Cancer Incidence

In the wake of reduced risk of prostate cancer, high-intensive endurance training of 5 weekly 120 min. sessions at 80% of the maximal oxygen uptake (VO_{2max}) seems to be appropriate owing to decreases of testosterone (T), lutropin (LH) and follitropine (FSH) levels and increases of sexual hormone-binding globulin (SHBG) being both associated with increased risk of prostate cancer at high concentration (T) resp. low concentration (SHBG) whereby immune defense could be adversely adjusted by too high intensity whereas resistance training needs to be furthermore examined because of an adverse effect on T, but a beneficial effect on immune defense.[148]

2.9.2 Sports & Exercise Training on Prostate Cancer Progression

A study recruited 26 patients with prostate cancer undergoing androgen deprivation therapy (ADT), carrying out a 6-month sports and exercise training intervention and being therefore randomly assigned into an endurance training group (EET) consisting of 5 weekly 60 min. sessions at 60% - 80% of the maximal heart rate (HR_{max}) and into a resistance training group (RET) comprising 5 weekly sessions of 10 strength exercises of the major muscle groups using resistance bands, a stability ball and an exercise mat and reached the conclusion that positive changes in adipokine levels and IGF-axis in respect to prostate cancer are mainly achieved by moderate-to-high intensity endurance training as compared with resistance training that may be pre-eminently coupled with healthy changes in physical fitness and body composition.[149] Another study recruited 10 healthy young male subjects aged 18 - 37, with 170 - 190 cm height, 58 - 82 kg of body weight and a median VO_{2max} of 3,7 L*min. All of them performed 20 min. of cycling at 125 W and 50% of the maximal oxygen uptake (VO_{2max}) on average whereupon the intensity was increased for 40 min. of cycling at 165 W and 65% of the maximal oxygen uptake (VO_{2max}) on average and so arrived at the result that 9 out of the afore-noted 10 subjects also showed an inhibitory effect on LNCaP cells being androgen-sensitive human prostate adenocarcinoma cells.[150] Another study incorporated 10 patients with prostate cancer undergoing androgen deprivation therapy (ADT) and performing a 20-week high-intensity resistance training of 2 weekly sessions of 8 exercises (chest press, leg press, lat pulldown, leg extension, shoulder press, leg curl, seated row, AB crunch) at 2 sets of 12 maximum repetitions in week 1 and 2, 3 sets of 10 maximum repetitions in week 3 and 4, 3 sets of 8 maximum repetitions in weeks 5 - 7, 4 sets of 6 maximum repetitions in weeks 8 - 10 as well as of 4 sets of 6 maximum repetitions of acute exercise bouts (chest press – seated row, squat, shoulder press – lat pulldown, leg press, triceps extension – biceps curl, leg extension – leg curl, upper rower dips, AB crunch – back extension) in weeks 11 - 20 with 60 - 90 sec. breaks between sets resp. 2 - 4 min. breaks between exercises each with the final outcome that T levels were slightly increased while SHBG and DHEA were significantly and prostate-specific antigen (PSA) slightly increased declaring the use of resistance training as adjuvant therapy for patients with prostate cancer has to be done with great care.[151] Generally speaking, "there is a growing body of epidemiological research suggesting that physical activity is protective against the development of prostate cancer" whereby the intensity and the type of sports and exercise training has to be contemplated because also after diagnosis, a higher level of sports and exercise training is statistically associated with reduced risk of prostate cancer progression.[152 153]

2.9.3 Sports & Exercise Training on Prostate Cancer Mortality

In general, "cardiac rehabilitation programs, which primarily utilize exercise, produce compelling and consistent clinical results. Randomized trials have repeatedly demonstrated that cardiac rehabilitation reduces the probability of suffering additional cardiac events and is associated with a broad range of benefits, including reduced mortality" whereat certain parameters increasing the risk of prostate cancer progression are inversely affected the most by moderate- to- high-intensity and prolonged endurance training in comparison with resistance training resp. shorter and/or low-to-moderate intensity endurance training.[154] A study involved 2.705 patients with non-metastatic prostate cancer, interviewed them to evaluate individual physical activity levels and accompanied them from 1990 - 2008 including 112 deaths because of prostate cancer whereby patients exercising 48 or more MET-hours per week (71 MET-hours per week on average), performing vigorous physical activity for 3 or more hours per week or performing non-vigorous physical activity for 10 or more hours per week showed the statistically best results as against lower volumes of the same intensity.[155] 1 MET (metabolic equivalent) is the rate of energy expenditure at rest whereby intensities of physical activities under 3 METs are considered to be as light, between 3 and 6

METs as moderate resp. above 6 METs as vigorous. MET-hours are calculated by METs times minutes of physical activities divided by 60.

2.9.4 Sports & Exercise Training on Palliative Care of Prostate Cancer

Concerning physical fitness and the quality of life in patients with prostate cancer in combination with endurance or resistance training, a combined supervised and self-directed sports and exercise training of endurance training embracing 30 min. sessions at 55% - 85% of the age-predicted maximal heart rate (HR_{max}) of 220 - age or 11 - 15 on the rate of perceived exertion (RPE) scale ranging from 6 (very light) - 20 (very hard) and a succeeding resistance training including 2 - 4 sets of body weight resistance and free weights involving large muscle groups at moderate-to-high intensity showed significant improvements in the quality of life, physical fitness and decreases in cancer-related fatigue.[156]

2.10 Cervical Cancer

Cervical cancer represents the cancer with the 10th highest mortality rate with 265.672 cancer deaths in 2012 worldwide by being the 4th most common and 4th deadliest cancer in 2012 among women with an incidence rate of 527.624 new cases as well as a mortality rate of 265.672 deaths in 2012 among women.[2] The most prevalent risk factor concerning the appearance of cervical cancer is the infection by the human papillomavirus (HPV). "HPV infections are the most common sexually transmitted infections globally. Genital HPV infection is associated with development of cervical cancer, cervical neoplasia, anogenital warts, and other anogenital cancers".[105] "Persistent HPV infection is a necessary, but not sufficient, cause of cervical cancer. High parity, … , poor sexual hygiene, … , multiple sexual partners, tobacco smoking, co-infection with human immunodeficiency virus, Herpes simplex virus type 2 and Chlamydia trachomatis, immunosuppression, oral contraceptive use and dietary deficiencies of vitamin A are all co-factors that are necessary for progression from cervical HPV infection to cancer".[106] Symptoms of cervical cancer may include vaginal discharge, postcoital bleeding, intermenstrual bleeding, heavier/longer menstrual periods, abdominal pain or dyspareunia.[107]

2.10.1 Sports & Exercise Training on Cervical Cancer Incidence

Referring to the impact of sports and exercise training on cervical cancer, a survey was conducted from 2006 - 2013 involving 1.125 women aged 18 - 65 years, not pregnant, not having a history of gynecological cancer, by questionnaire resulting in a lower risk for cervical cancer at 72 or more MET-hours per week as well as reduced risk of cervical intraepithelial neoplasia (CIN) at 38,5 - 72 resp. 72 or more MET-hours per week.[108] 1 MET (metabolic equivalent) is the rate of energy expenditure at rest whereby intensities of physical activities under 3 METs are considered to be as light, between 3 and 6 METs as moderate resp. above 6 METs as vigorous. MET-hours are calculated by METs times minutes of physical activities divided by 60. Although there is no clear evidence of a potential association between human papillomavirus (HPV) and sports and exercise training, HPV vaccine may be better accepted by women engaging in sports and exercise training in comparison with them with a lack of physical activity.[109] Increased levels or volumes of sports and exercise training are also associated with higher odds of pap screening, also called pap smear test, whereby the more the merrier takes effect herein.[110] "The Pap smear is used commonly as cytologic screening test for eradication of precancerous lesions" as well as "... performed with endocervical brush, fixed in 95% ethanol and stained by the Papanicolaou method".[111]

2.10.2 Sports & Exercise Training on Cervical Cancer Progression

A hardly verified trait could be the Lon protease being a human mitochondrial ATP-dependent stress protein that is up-regulated under stress conditions and also plays an important role in cervical cancer because of a significant increase of Lon protease levels that may promote cell proliferation and the cellular energy metabolism in cervical tissues whereas a down-regulation or inhibition of Lon protease can prevent or halt cell proliferation as well as modify the afore-remarked bioenergetic metabolism.[112] The Lon protease is effected by means of sports and exercise training due to the mere fact that in healthy people, Lon protease levels progressively decrease with advancing age while regular sports and exercise training seems to be able to prevent the age-related decline in Lon protease to avoid a restricted mitochondrial function.[113] But whether the Lon protease levels could be altered by sports and exercise training in patients with cervical cancer or for prevention of cervical cancer has to be explored yet owing to an increase of reactive oxygen species (ROS) production working mutagenic by a deficit in Lon protease in cervical

HeLa cells leading to elevated oxidative stress and less protection what can be counteracted by brief, moderate- to high-intensity endurance training at 70% - 85% of the maximal oxygen uptake (VO_{2max}) through increasing antioxidant defenses.[114][115]

2.11 Leukemia

Leukemia represents the cancer with the 11th highest mortality rate with 265.471 cancer deaths in 2012 worldwide by being the 11th most common and 9th deadliest cancer in 2012 among men resp. the 13th most common and 10th deadliest cancer in 2012 among women with an incidence rate of 200.676 new cases as well as a mortality rate of 151.321 deaths in 2012 among men resp. an incidence rate of 151.289 new cases as well as a mortality rate of 114.150 deaths in 2012 among women.[2] Leukemia represents an abnormally increased number of white blood cells whereby acute and chronic leukemia resp. myeloid and lymphocytic leukemia are distinguished. Leukemia is the most common type of childhood cancer including increasing leukemia rates associated with infections or incidence of immune-related illnesses such as allergy, asthma and type 1 diabetes in early or late childhood whereas risk factors in adults also include radiation, hydrocarbons, pesticides, alcohol use, cigarette smoking, illicit drug use or reproductive history as well as birth characteristics.[157][158] The most common symptom of acute leukemia appearing much earlier is fever whereas the most common symptom of chronic leukemia occurring to a subsequent date is a hepatosplenomegaly representing an enlargement of the liver and the spleen mainly because of an infection.[159]

2.11.1 Sports & Exercise Training on Leukemia Incidence

Due to a disturbance of the haematopoiesis, white blood cell (WBC) count abnormally increases while a shortage of fully functional white blood cells resp. declines of red blood cells and platelets are given whereby anemia can arise. A study recruited 26 men aged older than 65 years and allocated them into a control group (CG) with no history of regular exercise and into an exercise group (EG) with a history of sports and exercise training since adulthood for a mean of 4 weekly sessions of 60 - 120 min. per session and got to the result that WBC count was decreased in the EG as well as serological inflammatory and endocrine biomarkers were improved in the EG as compared to the CG.[160] Another study recruited 5 young active male subjects aged 25,4 years on average and exercising about 6 hours per week whereby all of them performed a high-intensity treadmill running test at 80% of the maximal oxygen uptake (VO_{2max}) being evaluated two weeks before by a progressive exercise test on ergometer and 2 weeks later, the same treadmill running test at 60% of the maximal oxygen uptake (VO_{2max}) whereby both tests began with 8 km/h, increased every 3 min. by 2 km/h. The final conclusion was that shortly after the test, only lymphocytes were reduced by moderate intensity whereby all other values showed increases whereas 1 hour after the test, lymphocytes were reduced under the baseline values by both tests while total WBC count was reduced under the blood volume by moderate-intensity resp. reduced as against shortly after the test values by high-intensity and granulocytes and monocytes were increased by both tests.[161]

2.11.2 Sports & Exercise Training on Palliative Care of Leukemia

A study involved 6 young patients aged 5 - 16 years with acute lymphocytic leukemia performing a 12-week in-hospital sports and exercise
training consisting of 2 weekly sessions of 10 min. warm-up on the
treadmill, 30 min. resistance training of 2 sets of 15 maximum repetitions in week 1 resp. 4 sets of 6 - 10 maximum repetitions throughout the
other weeks (bench press, leg press, lat pulldown, leg extension, seated
row) as well as 20 min. of treadmill running at 70% of the maximal oxygen uptake at the point of voluntary stopping (VO_{2peak}) whereby individual settings were evaluated by a treadmill test and by a 10-maximum
repetition test with the outcome that muscular strength and the quality of
life were improved.[162] Already a short 20 - 30 min. endurance training on
a cycle ergometer of an initial load of 25 W, increased by 10 W every 2
min. with the superior heart rate limit of 180 - age and performed three
times per week declines incidence rate of pneumonia and fever as potential risk factors of leukemia and common appearances during chemotherapy.[163]

2.12 Non-Hodgkin Lymphoma

Non-Hodgkin Lymphoma represents the cancer with the 12th highest
mortality rate with 199.670 cancer deaths in 2012 worldwide by being
the 9th most common and 11th deadliest cancer in 2012 among men resp.
the 11th most common and 12th deadliest cancer in 2012 among women
with an incidence rate of 217.643 new cases as well as a mortality rate of
115.404 deaths in 2012 among men resp. an incidence rate of 168.098
new cases as well as a mortality rate of 84.266 deaths in 2012 among

women.[2] Non-Hodgkin Lymphoma is a type of blood cancer originating from white blood cells called B- or T-lymphocytes being responsible for protecting everyone's immune system from endogenous or exogenous harmful cells or substances such as viruses and bacteria, but shall not be confused with Hodgkin Lymphoma whose difference is the occurrence of the Reed-Steinberg-Cell in the light microscopy in the biopsy. The most notable environmental risk factors include heavy alcohol consumption, heavy tobacco smoking, the excessive usage of hair dye products, UV- or ionizing radiation, diet including higher intake of fat and lower intake of fruits and vegetables, physical inactivity as well as chemical exposures whereas medical risk factors comprise infectious agents, obesity, autoimmune diseases, family history, blood transfusion, organ transplantation and medications such as statins or antibiotics.[184] The most common symptoms of Non-Hodgkin Lymphoma (NHL) are painless swellings in the neck, armpit and/or groin being body locations with groups of lymph nodes that produce and store cells against infections whereby other symptoms may include excessive nocturnal sweating, inexplicable wild fluctuations of body temperature as well as steep weight loss.[185]

2.12.1 Sports & Exercise Training on Non-Hodgkin Lymphoma Incidence

A study involved 1.030 NHL cases and 3.106 controls being interviewed by questionnaires about everyone's physical activity level, energy intake and BMI and observed from 1994 - 1997 with the final conclusion that those men exercising 19,1 or more MET-hours per week had odds ratios of 0,75 - 0,79 and those women exercising 15,2 or more MET-hours per week had ORs of 0,58 - 0,59 compared to those subjects exercising less 6,4 (men) resp. 6,1 (women) MET-hours per week.[186] 1 MET (metabolic equivalent) is the rate of energy expenditure at rest whereby intensities of physical activities under 3 METs are considered to be as light, between 3 and 6 METs as moderate resp. above 6 METs as vigorous. MET-hours are calculated by METs times minutes of physical activities divided by 60. Another, more recent study incorporating 950 NHL cases and 1.146 controls with a median age of 63 years being interviewed by questionnaire, too, arrived at the result that particularly BMI at young age, but also higher levels of physical activity may be factors to reduce risk of NHL pre-eminently in females while adult BMI and adult physical activity showed no association when men and women were pooled together although high-intensity sports and exercise training at young age may be suggested for reduced risk of NHL.[187] Another interesting approach would be the fact that low HDL-cholesterol levels seem to be associated with increased risk of NHL independent of other factors such as obesity or sports and exercise training usually affecting cholesterol whereby HDL-cholesterol levels can be significantly increased by combined endurance and resistance training of 3 weekly 60 min. sessions involving 20 min. of cycling at 60% of the maximal oxygen uptake at the point of voluntary stopping (VO_{2peak}) and whole-body exercises (bench press, shoulder press, biceps curls, triceps extensions, sit-ups and leg press) of 1 set of 10 - 15 maximum repetitions.[188 174]

2.12.2 Sports & Exercise Training on Palliative Care of Non-Hodgkin Lymphoma

The quality of life is positively associated with increased mental and physical health of NHL patients and survivors wherefore 319 NHL survivors with a median age of 59,8 years were interviewed and accompanied by questionnaire 2 - 5 years after diagnosis with the final outcome that those ones exercising 150 or more min. per week at moderate-to-high intensity reported mental and physical health benefits inclusive of decreased levels of depression and anxiety in comparison with those who were sedentary.[189] Relevant to the afore-mentioned topic of improved the quality of life, another study recruited 122 patients with lymphoma and randomly allocated them into a usual care group (UG) and a supervised endurance training group (AEG) performing a 12-week sports and exercise training program on a cycle ergometer of 3 weekly sessions of 15 - 20 min. for weeks 1 - 4 increased by 5 min. per week until 40 - 45 min. were reached at 60% of the maximal oxygen uptake at the point of voluntary stopping (VO_{2peak}) in week 1 increased by 5% per week until 75% was reached to investigate improvements in sleep quality by Pittsburgh Sleep Quality Index (PSQI) with the final result that the AEG may improve sleep quality merely from the point of view that patients already had poor sleep quality with or without adversely influencing clinical features including indolent, but not aggressive NHL at baseline.[190]

2.13 Brain Cancer

Brain Cancer represents the cancer with the 13th highest mortality rate with 189.382 cancer deaths in 2012 worldwide by being the 13th most common and 12th deadliest cancer in 2012 among men resp. the 16th most common and 13th deadliest cancer in 2012 among women with an incidence rate of 139.608 new cases as well as a mortality rate of 106.376 deaths in 2012 among men resp. an incidence rate of 116.605 new cases as well as a mortality rate of 83.006 deaths in 2012 among women.[2] There are many types of brain tumors, but the most common types comprise gliomas, meningiomas as well as pituitary and nerve sheath tumors whereby gliomas arising from glial cells being responsible for maintaining homeostasis, producing myelin as well as supplying neurons with oxygen and nutrients account for 80% of all malignant brain tumors.[191 192] When genetic risk factors are excluded, proven environmental risk factors merely include high-dose ionizing radiation while heavy alcohol consumption, chemical agents, cellphones, head traumas or injuries, infections, occupational exposures to rubber or vinyl chloride and tobacco smoking may also play a role, which have not been proven yet. Symptoms of brain cancer embrace headache, memory loss, cognitive changes, motor deficit, language deficit and seizures, but also personality change, visual problems, consciousness change, nausea, vomiting, sensory deficit as well as clearly visible papilledema.[193]

2.13.1 Sports & Exercise Training on Brain Cancer Incidence

A study was concerned with glioma being the most common form of brain cancer and detected that high-, moderate- and/or light-intensity physical activity of at least 51,6 MET-hours per week between ages 15 and 18 was inversely associated with glioma risk whereas physical activity in adults was not affected by that whereby BMI was also solely associated with reduced risk of glioma during adolescence, but not in adulthood.[194] 1 MET (metabolic equivalent) is the rate of energy expenditure at rest whereby intensities of physical activities under 3 METs are considered to be as light, between 3 and 6 METs as moderate resp. above 6 METs as vigorous. MET-hours are calculated by METs times minutes of physical activities divided by 60. Another interesting subject area could be a potential connection between brain cancer and stroke due to stroke-like syndromes such as progressive weakness of the right upper and lower limbs, headache, blurring of vision or slurring has already been able to be observed in the past.[195] Therefore, resistance training to increase independence in daily activities, flexibility training to increase range of motion, balance training to improve coordination and endurance training of moderate intensity to increase physical capacity and reduce risk of cardiovascular diseases should be performed at least three times per week for 20 - 60 min. each session to provide protective benefits in the prevention and recurrence of stroke or to improve functional outcomes in stroke survivors.[196]

2.13.2 Sports & Exercise Training on Brain Cancer Mortality

Concerning a potential association between sports and exercise training and reduced risk of brain cancer, a study recruited 111.266 runners and 42.136 walkers and accompanied them 11,7 years on average where 110 brain cancer deaths were identified and finally arrived at the result that runners and walkers exercising 1,8 or more MET-hours per day had a

42,5% lower risk of brain cancer mortality.[197] Another study attending to glioma involved 243 patients with grade 3 - 4 recurrent malignant glioma primarily completing a questionnaire to assess physical activity levels, subsequently performing a 6-minute walk test (6MWT) and lastly being followed up with the final outcome that those patients exercising 9 or more MET-hours per week averagely survived 21,84 months and also had a much higher survival probability compared to those patients exercising less than 9 MET-hours per week with a median survival of 13,03 months and a much smaller survival probability whereas better or weaker outcomes in the 6MWT seemed to have no influence on survival time or survival probability of those patients.[198]

2.13.3 Sports & Exercise Training on Palliative Care of Brain Cancer

Sports and exercise training can also improve functional outcomes of brain cancer patients what was illustrated by a study containing 75 brain cancer patients who underwent surgery and 75 patients who were affected by a stroke whereby all of them participated in a 2-year sports and exercise training program of 6 weekly 60 min. sessions including 10 min. stretching and 10 min. strengthening of the whole body, 15 min. strengthening of the upper limb and/or hands, 10 min. balance exercises in sitting and standing positions as well as 15 min. ground-floor walking with and without assistance with additional benefits for the quality of life.[199]

2.14 Bladder Cancer

Bladder Cancer represents the cancer with the 14th highest mortality rate with 165.084 cancer deaths in 2012 worldwide by being the 7th most common and 10th deadliest cancer in 2012 among men resp. the 19th most common and 17th deadliest cancer in 2012 among women with an incidence rate of 330.380 new cases as well as a mortality rate of 123.051 deaths in 2012 among men resp. an incidence rate of 99.413 new cases as well as a mortality rate of 42.033 deaths in 2012 among women.[2] The most important risk factor for the development of bladder cancer is an exposure to aromatic amines being increasingly used as starting products for the production of pharmaceutical substances, pesticides, synthetic material or dyestuff whereas other well-known risk factors include tobacco smoking and arsenic in drinking water.[177] The most prevalent clinical symptoms contain haematuria in about 65% of men resp. 68% of women, nocturia in about 57% of men resp. 66% of women, urgency in about 61% of men resp. 47% of women and dysuria in about 32% of men resp. 44% of women.[178]

2.14.1 Sports & Exercise Training on Bladder Cancer Incidence

Regarding a potential association between sports and exercise training and reduced bladder cancer risk, a study recruited 803 Caucasian bladder cancer patients and 803 healthy Caucasian subjects in 1999 and obtained information by questionnaire about everyone's approximate daily energy intake and physical activity level being calculated by MET. The final outcome indicated that intensive physical activity of 25 or more METs combined with a medium daily energy intake of 1738 - 2312 kcal achieved the best results and may have protective effects with an odds ratio of 0,76 whereby also people with high energy intake of more than 2312 kcal/d, low physical activity of less than 9 METs and 7 or more unfavorable genotypes may have 21,93-fold increased risk for bladder cancer as against those with low energy intake of less than 1738 kcal/d, intensive physical activity of 25 or more METs and a low number of unfavorable genotypes.[179] 1 MET (metabolic equivalent) is the rate of energy expenditure at rest whereby intensities of physical activities under 3 METs are considered to be as light, between 3 and 6 METs as moderate resp. above 6 METs as vigorous. MET-hours are calculated by METs times minutes of physical activities divided by 60. As opposed to that, another prospective study containing 471.760 men and women from the USA found no correlation between any levels of physical activity and reduced bladder carcinogenesis whereat obesity was modestly linked to risk of bladder cancer.[180] All in all, behavioral and lifestyle factors such as pelvic floor muscle exercises can significantly increase bladder health by improving contraction, relaxation and resistance of the urinary bladder as well as sports and exercise training could be a suitable adjuvant therapy due to a high coincidence of bladder and prostate cancer that might be outlined by a common and similar carcinogenic pathway.[181] [182]

2.14.2 Sports & Exercise Training on Palliative Care of Bladder Cancer

However, sports and exercise training is also positively associated with health benefits in bladder cancer survivors including increased the quality of life and reduced cancer-related fatigue what could also be illustrated by a study containing 525 bladder cancer survivors whereby appropriate sports and exercise training guidelines cannot be adhered by a lot of bladder cancer patients especially when they undergo cystectomy what in turn should be contemplated.[183]

2.15 Ovarian Cancer

Ovarian cancer represents the cancer with the 15th highest mortality rate with 151.917 cancer deaths in 2012 worldwide by being the 7th most common and 8th deadliest cancer in 2012 among women with an incidence rate of 238.719 new cases as well as a mortality rate of 151.917 deaths in 2012 among women.[2] Ovarian cancer emanates from epithelial tissue whereby serous cystomas, mucinous cystomas, endometroid tumors, clear-cell tumors and other unclassified or malignant tumors can occur.[135] "The most significant risk factor, hereditary ovarian cancer syndrome, increases the possibility of developing ovarian cancer by 25% - 50%. Women have a 4% - 5% increased risk if a single family member was diagnosed with ovarian cancer, whereas those with two or more family members have a 7% increased risk. Other hereditary syndromes are site-specific ovarian cancer, breast-ovarian cancer, and the family cancer syndrome. Breast-ovarian cancer syndrome causes almost 90% of hereditary ovarian cancers and usually is associated with mutations in BRCA1 or BRCA2 genes. Hormonal risk factors include nulliparity, infertility, early menarche, late menopause, and endometriosis. Environmental and lifestyle risk factors are diet and obesity. Perineal talc exposure also is a risk factor …".[135] The most substantial symptoms that should be paid attention to are abdominal swelling, pelvic pain, abdominal bloating, but also vaginal bleeding, vaginal discharge, altered bowel habits and indigestion.[136]

2.15.1 Sports & Exercise Training on Ovarian Cancer Incidence

An association between physical activity and reduced risk of ovarian cancer is slightly given by exercising 23 or more MET-hours per week at high intensity.[137] Another study also came to the final conclusion that women exercising 31,5 or more MET-hours per week had got a 27% reduced risk of ovarian cancer than women exercising nothing as well as light and moderate physical activity levels were not associated with reduced ovarian cancer risk resp. longer sitting of 6 or more hours per day was associated with higher risk of ovarian cancer as against sitting of less than 3 hours per day.[138] 1 MET (metabolic equivalent) is the rate of energy expenditure at rest whereby intensities of physical activities under 3 METs are considered to be as light, between 3 and 6 METs as moderate resp. above 6 METs as vigorous. MET-hours are calculated by METs times minutes of physical activities divided by 60. Regarding hormonal influences, the Gonadotropin-releasing hormone (GnRH) controlling the secretion of Follitropine (FSH) and Lutropin (LH) from the adenohypophysis and hence possibly playing a role in ovarian cancer by changing signaling pathways, affecting gene expression or increasing tumor cell proliferation are highly expressed in epithelial ovarian cancer.[139] Because of the fact that, in turn FSH and LH concurrently stimulate the secretion and expression of sexual hormones from the ovaries, we could just take it as read that those sexual hormones are also highly expressed in ovarian cancer. Confirmation by current literature is scarce, but BRCA1/BRCA2 mutation carriers showing higher levels of estrogen and estradiol whereby high estradiol levels is associated with higher risk in ovarian carcinogenesis in such women.[140] A study reached the conclusion of decreased levels of estrone, estradiol, testosterone and androstenedione by doing combined reduced-calorie weight loss diet being comprised of a daily energy intake of 1.200 - 2.000 kcal including 30% or less from fat and moderate- to vigorous-intensity endurance training on the treadmill consisting of a 12-month sports and exercise training intervention of 5 weekly sessions of 225 min. per week at an intensity of 70% - 85% of the maximal heart rate (HR_{max}) measured by a maximal graded treadmill test by previously allocating 439 postmenopausal women aged 50 - 75 into 4 groups (control, only diet, only exercise, diet + exercise) and comparing the outcomes.[48]

2.15.2 Sports & Exercise Training on Ovarian Cancer Progression

Among the genes showing the greatest up-regulation in ovarian cancer and high-risk population is interleukin-8 (IL-8) whereas sports and exercise training is able to increase IL-8 levels in healthy individuals and decrease IL-8 levels in patients with metabolic syndrome doing a 3-month combined training consisting of 40% endurance training of walking, jogging or cycling at 80% of the maximal heart rate (HR_{max}) and 60% resistance training of 15 - 20 repetitions each exercise three times per week lasting 45 - 60 min. each whereby also a 12-week moderate-intensity endurance training consisting of 3 weekly sessions of 40 - 50 min. of walking at 50% - 60% of the heart rate reserve (HR_{res}) being calculated by maximal heart rate minus resting heart rate also significantly decreases IL-8.[141 90 91] Also endothelin-1 (ET-1), a protein and vasoconstrictor being produced by vascular endothelial cells, is highly overexpressed in primary and metastatic ovarian cancer whereas a 24-week sports and exercise training intervention conducted four times per week of mere endurance training involving 60-min. brisk walking at 60% - 70% of the maximal heart rate (HR_{max}) or combined endurance and resistance training of a shortened 20-min. brisk walking workout at the same heart rate and of 30-min. resistance training of the upper arm, chest, waist, abdomen and legs at 2 - 4 sets of 15 - 20 repetitions each decreases levels of ET-1.[142][143]

2.15.3 Sports & Exercise Training on Palliative Care of Ovarian Cancer

The intensity of sports and exercise training should be upheld high to increase the benefits in relation to ovarian cancer whereas also a 24-week light- to moderate-intensity endurance training of brisk walking at 60% - 70% of the maximal heart rate (HR_{max}) or at 4 - 7 on a 10-point rate of perceived exertion (RPE) scale ranging from 1 (very light) – 10 (very hard) combined with 10 strength exercises (squats, push-ups, seated row, hamstring curls, lateral raises, triceps extension, biceps curls, upright rows, crunches, hip extension) of 2 sets of 8 - 12 repetitions each exercise comprising 3 - 5 weekly sessions lasting 30 - 60 min. each session significantly increases physical fitness and the quality of life in patients with ovarian cancer.[144] Increased moderate to vigorous physical activity is associated with increased quality of life and increased physical well-being during chemotherapy being in turn a prognostic indicator for overall survival in women undergoing chemotherapy for ovarian cancer.[145]

2.16 Kidney Cancer

Kidney Cancer represents the cancer with the 16th highest mortality rate with 143.406 cancer deaths in 2012 worldwide by being the 10th most common and 13th deadliest cancer in 2012 among men resp. the 15th most common and 16th deadliest cancer in 2012 among women with an incidence rate of 213.924 new cases as well as a mortality rate of 90.802 deaths in 2012 among men resp. an incidence rate of 123.936 new cases as well as a mortality rate of 52.604 deaths in 2012 among women.[2] Well-established risk factors except genetic factors include tobacco smoking, obesity and hypertension resp. risk factors having less evidence range from diabetes mellitus to reproductive and hormonal factors primarily in women as well as physical inactivity and occupational exposure to industrial chemical agents Trichloroethylene (TCE).[200] On the other hand, primary symptoms embrace hematuria, bone pain combined with general pain and lingering cough resp. secondary symptoms comprise shortness of breath, continued fever, weight loss, lack of energy as well as weariness.[201]

2.16.1 Sports & Exercise Training on Kidney Cancer Incidence

In the past, high-quality studies noticed that high-level physical activity is inversely associated with increased risk of kidney cancer whereby other well-established or potential risk factors were not observed.[202] A study observed 289.503 men and 192.883 women aged 50 - 71 years from 1995 - 2003 and thereby determined everyone's physical activity level during adolescence and nowadays by baseline questionnaire by information of how often they exercised at least 20 min. between ages 15 - 18 and exercise at least 20 min. in the present that causes sweating, increased breathing and/or increased heart rate whereat 929 men and 309 women were diagnosed with kidney cancer and the final outcome showed the most benefits of physical activity for reduced kidney cancer risk by exercising three - four times per week during adolescence, 5 or more times per week in the present and regularly climbing stairs or hills or lifting light weights.[203] Another study detected that people with highly above-average IGF-I levels had a significantly reduced risk to develop kidney cancer in comparison with those having highly below-average IGF-I levels as well as a non-significantly positive association for higher IGFBP-3 levels in respect to kidney cancer whereby the investigated group merely consisted of male smokers aged 50 - 69 years.[204] On the other hand, resistance training what was tested in 11 healthy individuals can significantly increase IGF-I levels. Those ones performed 3 repetitions of knee extension under alternating concentric and eccentric conditions at 40% resp. 110% of the 1 repetition maximum whereby higher increases of IGF-I levels were ascertained during the trial with 40% of the 1 repetition maximum whereas neither a short-term high-intensity endurance training (HIT) nor a high-volume endurance training (HVT) affected IGF-I levels, but solely a HIT also significantly increased IGFBP-3 levels what can be seen as counterproductive for risk reduction of kidney cancer.[205 206] IGF-I is a protein being secreted by the liver after the stimulation of somatotropin representing the human growth hormone (HGH) and being responsible for the growth process of all types of tissues whereas IGFBP-3 binds to IGF-I in the liver and promotes the stimulation of somatotropin. Another study interviewed 91.820 subjects to assess everyone's physical activity level and accompanied them between 1991 and 1993 resp. between 1998 and 1999 as well as arrived at the result that also endurance training in the form of walking and running 12,6 or more MET-hours per week may be positively associated with reduced risk of kidney cancer.[207] 1 MET (metabolic equivalent) is the rate of energy expenditure at rest whereby intensities of physical activities under 3 METs are considered to be as light, between 3 and 6 METs as moderate resp. above 6 METs as vigorous. MET-hours are calculated by METs times minutes of physical activities divided by 60. Because of the fact that hypertension is a well-established risk factor for kidney cancer, prescribed sports and exercise training should contain 2 - 3 weekly sessions of resistance training of 10 exercises per session with 8 - 25 repetitions at about 60% of the 1 repetition maximum and 3 weekly sessions of endurance training of at least 40 min. per session at about 65% of the heart rate reserve (HR_{res}) being calculated by maximal heart rate minus resting heart rate to decrease hypertension and even-handedly the risk of kidney cancer.[208] Also obesity and logically metabolic syndrome are both associated with increased risk of kidney cancer, whereby a combination of moderate-intensity endurance training having the much greater energy expenditure with resistance training having much greater benefits in improvements of lipid profiles and insulin resistance during additional dietary energy restriction, which is more effective in promoting weight loss, preventing obesity and reducing the risk of kidney cancer.[209]

2.17 Gallbladder Cancer

Gallbladder Cancer represents the cancer with the 16th highest mortality rate with 143.406 cancer deaths in 2012 worldwide by being the 15th most common and 14th deadliest cancer in 2012 among men resp. the

18th most common and 14th deadliest cancer in 2012 among women with
an incidence rate of 76.844 new cases as well as a mortality rate of
60.339 deaths in 2012 among men resp. an incidence rate of 101.257
new cases as well as a mortality rate of 82.484 deaths in 2012 among
women.[2] The only well-established risk factor of gallbladder cancer is
the appearance of gallstones whereat gallstones alone merely account for
a small percentage for gallbladder cancer development whereas other
potential accompanying risk factors obesity or cholecystitis together with
cholelithiasis also play a major role to increase the risk.[218] Other non-
specific risk factors may include abnormal pancreaticobiliary duct junc-
tion, heavy red meat consumption, heavy tobacco smoking, chronic biliary infections, porcelain gallbladder as well as diabetes mellitus whereas
symptoms are hard to perceive, but may comprise abdominal pain, unexpected and sudden weight loss, continued or fulminating fever as well as
jaundice.[219]

2.17.1 Sports & Exercise Training on Gallbladder Cancer Incidence

Concerning a potential association between physical activity and hepatobiliary cancers, a study involved 507.897 participants aged 50 - 71 by
completing a questionnaire of how often physical activity that increases
respiration, heart rate or perspiration is done whereby never (1), rarely
(2), one to three times per month (3), one to two times per week (4),
three to four times per week (5) and five or more times per week (6)
were the options listed with the final outcome that five or more times per
week may have the potential of reducing the risk of gallbladder cancer.[67]
One reason can be that high-level physical activity also contributing to
lower biliary cholesterol levels and preventing cholesterol to precipitate
in the bile reduces the risk of gallstones by up to 70% after

5 years and by up to 30% after 14 years compared to low-level physical activity being associated with gallstone formation.[220][221] A combined endurance and resistance training and concurrent dietary energy restriction is able to avoid obesity and metabolic syndrome by interval training of 4 x 4 min. at 90% of the maximal heart rate (HR_{max}) with 3 min. active recoveries at 70% of the maximal heart rate (HR_{max}) in between with 10 min. warm-up and 5 min. cool down as well as continuous moderate endurance training (CME) of 47 min. at 70% of the maximal heart rate (HR_{max}) can help to reduce risk of gallbladder cancer.[214]

2.18 Multiple Myeloma

Multiple myeloma represents the cancer with the 18th highest mortality rate with 80.019 cancer deaths in 2012 worldwide by being the 17th most common and 15th deadliest cancer in 2012 among men resp. the 20th most common and 18th deadliest cancer in 2012 among women with an incidence rate of 62.469 new cases as well as a mortality rate of 43.091 deaths in 2012 among men resp. an incidence rate of 51.782 new cases as well as a mortality rate of 36.928 deaths in 2012 among women.[2] Multiple myeloma represents a type of cancer where the number of malignant plasma cells is progressively increased in the bone marrow, bones or other tissues whereby concurrently large amounts of paraproteins being disease-causing are also produced while healthy plasma cells being usually responsible for immune defense and the production of antibodies are suppressed and healthy defensive proteins are insufficiently produced.[222] Risk factors of multiple myeloma are generally unknown whereat a BMI above 30, walking less than 30 min. per day, discontent in personal and/or occupational lives as well as history of peptic ulcers could contribute to increase risk of multiple myeloma.[223] The most important symptoms of multiple myeloma are the CRAB symptoms including hypercalcemia, renal insufficiency, anemia and bone lesions whereby also non-CRAB symptoms such as infections, cryoglobulinemia, secondary gout, leukemia, hemorrhage, systemic symptoms (e.g. fever, weight loss), amyloidosis, hyperviscocity syndrome, neuropathy (e.g. nerve root compression) or extramedullary involvement could also play a minor role.[224]

2.18.1 Sports & Exercise Training on Multiple Myeloma Incidence

A study containing 121.700 women aged 30 - 55 years and 51.529 men aged 40 - 75 years being followed from 1976 (women) resp. 1986 (men) until multiple myeloma diagnosis, death or 2002 and being also interviewed by questionnaires every 2 years from baseline about their BMIs and physical activity levels whereby a BMI above 30 was most badly associated with increased risk of multiple myeloma while an inverse association of physical activity in respect to multiple myeloma risk was merely achieved in women exercising 2 or more hours per week without a statistically significant risk reduction in men.[225] So sports and exercise training seems to be appropriate at preventing too high BMIs whereas a solely protective effect remains unclear. But also CRAB symptoms, the most common symptoms in multiple myeloma, can be partially trained and improved by sports and exercise training. A decrease in intracellular calcium and an increase in parathormone (PTH) regulating the calcium level and maybe also helping bone metabolism is achieved by just a single bout of sports and exercise training whereby 45 min. endurance training sessions at already 50% of the maximal oxygen uptake (VO_{2max}) is recommended every 72 hours because of reduced intracellular calcium, increased PTH as well as improved calcium homeostasis.[226] Renal insufficiency can also be prevented by regular sports and exercise training due to positively influencing blood pressure resp. reducing excess body weight, insulin resistance and vessel rigidity as potential risk factors whereby at least a moderate endurance training of 30 min. and a moderate resistance training of 12 - 15 repetitions per set should be performed.[227] Sports and exercise training also increases total hemoglobin mass and consequently counteracts anemia representing the decrease of red blood cells by stimulating erythropoiesis and subsequently increasing the amount of oxygen by higher demands of working skeletal muscles to optimize microcirculation and to provide the vasodilator nitric oxide.[228] Concerning the prevention of bone lesions, high-impact type of sports and exercise training improves bone mineral density (BMD), bone mineral content (BMC) as well as bone strength what should be promoted at young age, too.[229] Another study involving 135 patients with multiple myeloma being randomly allocated into a usual care group (UG) and an exercise group (EG) of a combined endurance training comprising 20 min. of daily walking and a moderate resistance training was concerned with the impacts of sports and exercise training and additional erythropoietin (EPO) therapy three times per week and found out that the EG with EPO therapy reduced the number of red blood cell transfusions and simultaneously increased cardiorespiratory fitness in those patients.[230] Another interesting factor that should be taken into consideration is that the activity of natural killer cells being responsible for killing cancer, tumor and virus-infected cells is also increased during recovery of a 30 min. endurance training slightly below or above the anaerobic threshold (AT) in 16 healthy cyclists aged 18 - 50 years on average being previously tested in a lactate threshold test including 3 min. incremental stages with increases of 20 - 25 W per stage.[231]

2.19 Endometrial Cancer

Endometrial Cancer represents the cancer with the 19th highest mortality rate with 76.160 cancer deaths in 2012 worldwide by being the 6th most common and 15th deadliest cancer in 2012 among women with an incidence rate of 319.605 new cases as well as a mortality rate of 76.160 deaths in 2012 among women.[2] A review of the literature showed that the risk of endometrial cancer is increased by older age, early menarche and late menopause, obesity, family history whereby close family members are pre-eminently affected, radiation exposure, increased estrogen and decreased progesterone levels as well as infertility particularly in the presence of Polycystic Ovary Syndrome (POS) representing an endocrine disorder leading to high androgen levels and being mostly diagnosed in obese women.[210] The most common symptom is abnormal uterine and/or irregular menstrual bleeding being considered a warning sign and a high-risk factor for malignancy in endometrial cancer.[211]

2.19.1 Sports & Exercise Training on Endometrial Cancer Incidence

A study lasting from 2002 - 2006 involved 542 endometrial cancer cases and 1.032 controls being interviewed about their physical activity levels with the final outcome that light-intensity physical activity of less than 3

METs being performed more than 21,6 hours per week had the best OR of 0,68 and the most benefits in reducing endometrial cancer risk.[212] 1 MET (metabolic equivalent) is the rate of energy expenditure at rest whereby intensities of physical activities under 3 METs are considered to be as light, between 3 and 6 METs as moderate resp. above 6 METs as vigorous. MET-hours are calculated by METs times minutes of physical activities divided by 60. Internally inconsistent, most of the studies in the recent past showed apparent risk reduction by doing moderate-to-vigorous physical activity that may complement increasing daily sitting time that progressively increases the risk of endometrial cancer.[213] Combined endurance and resistance training and concurrent dietary energy restriction can prevent obesity being a well-established risk factor and metabolic syndrome whereby regarding endurance training, interval training (AIT) consisting of 4 x 4 min. intervals at 90% of the maximal heart rate (HR_{max}) with 3 min. active recoveries at 70% of the maximal heart rate (HR_{max}) in between with 10 min. warm-up and 5 min. cool down as well as continuous moderate endurance training (CME) of 47 min. at 70% of the maximal heart rate (HR_{max}) can be applied at least three times per week whereat both types were effective at reducing body weight and body fat with light advantages for CME while AIT showed better outcomes in insulin signaling and reducing blood glucose, but also conversely in decreasing lipogenesis, which was tested in 32 metabolic syndrome patients being randomly allocated into an AIT, a CME and a control group.[214] A potential connection between endometrial and breast cancer is the increased risk of both cancer types by increased levels of estrogen. Because estrogen at high levels significantly increase the risk of endometrial cancer 5-fold and beyond whereby a difference exists by various risk factor levels in progesterone.[215] Therefore 10 healthy, premenopausal and eumenorrheic women aged 25 - 35 years and classified at high risk of breast cancer, were recruited in a study lasting 7 menstrual cycles and consisting of a home-based sports and exercise training program on a treadmill altogether lasting 12 weeks and starting after the 2nd menstrual cycle whereby 3 women did not remain until completion of the study. Each participant had to perform 3 weekly sessions of overall 150 min. in weeks 1 and 2, 200 min. in weeks 3 and 4, 225 min. in weeks 5 and 6, 250 min. in weeks 7 and 8, 275 min. in weeks 10 and 11 as well as 300 min. in weeks 11 and 12 whereby one session had to last at least 15 min., but was not allowed to exceed 100 min. including an intensity of 80% - 85% of the maximal heart rate (HR_{max}) being primarily evaluated by an incremental treadmill test with the result of lower total estrogen and total progesterone levels whereas the menstrual cycle length was not influenced.[42] "Hyper-insulinemia, low free IGF-I, and high estradiol levels may together account for a substantial proportion of endometrial cancers because they are each common exposures with moderate to strong associations with the risk for endometrial cancer".[216] Another study got to the outcome of reduced levels of estrone, estradiol, testosterone and androstenedione that may reduce risk of endometrial cancer by doing combined reduced-calorie weight loss diet being comprised of a daily energy intake of 1.200 to 2.000 kcal including 30% or less from fat and moderate- to vigorous-intensity endurance training on the treadmill consisting of a 12-month sports and exercise training intervention of 5 weekly sessions of 225 min. per week at an intensity of 70% - 85% of the maximal heart rate (HR_{max}) measured by a maximal graded treadmill test by previously allocating 439 postmenopausal women aged 50 - 75 into 4 groups (control, only diet, only exercise, diet + exercise) and comparing the outcomes.[48] IGF-I levels can in turn be significantly increased by resistance training at low- to high-intensity of the 1 repetition maximum whereas neither a short-term high-intensity endurance training nor a high-volume endurance training affected IGF-I levels whereby potential alterations in IGF-I levels should also be verified after high-intensity endurance training.[205 206]

2.19.2 Sports & Exercise Training on Endometrial Cancer Mortality

Obesity is a well-established risk factor whereby in patients suffering from endometrial cancer, the endometrial cancer-specific mortality is still much higher than the all-cause mortality for progressively elevated BMI levels in comparison with normal BMI levels.[217] As mentioned before, combined interval training of 4 x 4 min. intervals at 90% of the maximal heart rate (HR_{max}) with 3 min. active recoveries at 70% of the maximal heart rate (HR_{max}) in between with 10 min. warm-up and 5 min. cool down as well as continuous moderate exercise (CME) of 47 min. at 70% of the maximal heart rate (HR_{max}) being applied at least three times per week and simultaneous dietary energy restriction can prevent obesity with slight advantages for CME in reducing body fat while AIT showed better outcomes in insulin signaling and reducing blood glucose, but also conversely in decreasing lipogenesis.[214]

2.20 Skin Cancer

Skin Cancer excluding non-melanoma skin cancer represents the cancer with the 20th highest mortality rate with 55.488 cancer deaths in 2012 worldwide by being the 14th most common and 16th deadliest cancer in

2012 among men resp. the 17th most common and 20th deadliest cancer in 2012 among women with an incidence rate of 120.649 new cases as well as a mortality rate of 31.390 deaths in 2012 among men resp. an incidence rate of 111.481 new cases as well as a mortality rate of 24.098 deaths in 2012 among women.[2] Melanoma skin cancer represents the most dangerous type of skin cancer being caused by melanocytes that are cells being responsible for the production of skin pigments called melanin whereas non-melanoma skin cancer being subdivided into basal cell carcinoma (BCC) and squamous cell carcinoma (SCC) represents the generally most common type of cancer worldwide with an estimated incidence rate of 2 – 3 million new cases per year.[232] The most important risk factor of skin cancer is UV radiation whereby the role of other factors such as human papillomavirus, HIV/AIDS and Non-Hodgkin lymphoma, ionizing radiation or environmental risk factors including medication use, tobacco smoking, food consumption or stress are only widely supposed, but unproven.[233 234] Symptoms of melanoma skin cancer are moles that get bigger, change shape and/or color, loses symmetry, are painful, are bleeding and/or look inflamed whereas symptoms of non-melanoma skin cancer can appear as a spot or sore that does not heal within 4 weeks and/or continues to hurt for more than 4 weeks with an ulcer, which can arise, whereby BCC looks like a small, slow growing, shiny, pink or red lump and SCC looks like a pink lump.[235 236]

2.20.1 Sports & Exercise Training on Skin Cancer

In current studies, sports and exercise training is not in the least associated with reduced risk of each type of skin cancer whereas exercise-induced immunosuppression during strong sun exposure without or with too less sun protection can additionally increase the risk of melanoma and non-melanoma skin cancer, so that midday sun should be avoided and sufficient sun protection should be considered during the warm season.[237]

2.21 Thyroid Cancer

Thyroid Cancer represents the cancer with the 21st highest mortality rate with 39.771 cancer deaths in 2012 worldwide by being the 16th most common and 19th deadliest cancer in 2012 among men resp. the 8th most common and 19th deadliest cancer in 2012 among women with an incidence rate of 68.179 new cases as well as a mortality rate of 12.626 deaths in 2012 among men resp. an incidence rate of 229.923 new cases as well as a mortality rate of 27.145 deaths in 2012 among women.[2] Potential risk factors of thyroid cancer include exposure to ionizing radiation, iodine deficiency, high levels of nitrate, environmental pollution, high levels of thyroid-stimulating hormone (TSH) stimulating thyroxine and triiodthyronine in turn stimulating energy metabolism in most tissues, and thyroiditis.[248] The most common symptoms of thyroid cancer comprise a lump at the base of the neck or elsewhere in the neck, a hoarse voice lasting for more than a few weeks and/or a sore throat with difficulty in swallowing that does not get better whereby unusual symptoms such as diarrhea or flushing face could also, but rarely appear because of a too high level of calcitonin representing a hormone being produced by the parathyroid glands and regulating the calcium balance.[249]

2.21.1 Sports & Exercise Training on Thyroid Cancer Incidence

Current studies investigating large groups of males and females over a long period of time did not find any association between increased physical activity levels and reduced risk of thyroid cancer whereby also diabetes history was not linked to increased risk.[250][251] Whereas, on the other hand, another recent study involving 116.939 women aged 22 - 79 years being followed from 1995/1996 until 2009 and interviewed about everyone's participation level in moderate- to high-intensity physical activity in the last 3 years whereby 275 diagnosis of papillary thyroid cancer being the most common type of thyroid cancer appeared and the final conclusion was that long-term moderate- to high-intensity physical activity of at least 16,5 MET-hours per week as well as a BMI under 25 was strongly associated with reduced risk of papillary thyroid cancer mainly spreading to the lymph nodes in the neck.[252] 1 MET (metabolic equivalent) is the rate of energy expenditure at rest whereby intensities of physical activities under 3 METs are considered to be as light, between 3 and 6 METs as moderate resp. above 6 METs as vigorous. MET-hours are calculated by METs times minutes of physical activities divided by 60.

2.21.2 Sports & Exercise Training on Thyroid Cancer Progression

An option for a positive impact could be that most of the patients with papillary thyroid cancer show low levels of STAT3 being a gene responsible for producing proteins taking part in essential chemical signaling ways within cells and leading to increases in glucose consumption, lactate production and expression of Hypoxia-inducible factor 1 (HIF1) promote aerobic glycolysis and tumor proliferation while STAT3 activation seems to be a negative regulator of aerobic glycolysis and thyroid tumor growth.[253] The fact that already a single bout of intense resistance training of 12 maximum repetitions with concentric and eccentric phases significantly increases STAT3 signalling could also underline or be an indicator for the beneficial role of sports and exercise training to reduce risk of papillary thyroid cancer whereby it was only tested in untrained, but active males on knee extension and flexion while STAT3 increases were much more significant after sports and exercise training in older people in comparison to younger ones.[254 255]

2.22 Kaposi Sarcoma

Kaposi Sarcoma represents the cancer with the 22nd highest mortality rate with 26.974 cancer deaths in 2012 worldwide by being represented the 20th most common and 17th deadliest cancer in 2012 among men resp. the 22nd most common and 22nd deadliest cancer in 2012 among women with an incidence rate of 29.022 new cases as well as a mortality rate of 17.358 deaths in 2012 among men resp. an incidence rate of 15.225 new cases as well as a mortality rate of 9.616 deaths in 2012 among women.[2] Kaposi sarcoma (KS) emanates from cells lining lymph or blood vessels being infected by human herpesvirus 8 (HHV8) causing a high division rate and longer preservation of those cells obviously leading to the emergence of cancer cells and usually appears on the skin or on mucosal surfaces, but other body parts such as lymph nodes or the digestive tract can also be affected whereby purple, red or brown blotches often occur on the skin of the legs and face resulting in skin lesions in those affected areas, but also metastases can often be found being able to cause breathing problems when the lungs are concerned resp. gastrointestinal bleeding when the digestive tract are affected.[243] As a consequence, the infection with HHV8 is a requirement for the development of KS, but does not automatically brings about the emergence of KS while other additional risk factors such as AIDS/HIV or immunodeficiency may also play a notable role.[244]

2.22.1 Sports & Exercise Training on Kaposi Sarcoma Incidence

There is no clear state of evidence of a possible association between physical activity and reduced risk of KS. An approach could also be the inhibition or decrease of viral interleukin-6 (vIL-6) representing an inflammatory marker, which is released at the place of inflammation due to high expressions of vIL-6 in HHV-8-associated malignancies including KS that can be optimally down-regulated by high-level physical activity of 50% of the maximum workload including endurance and/or resistance training of long duration of 1 - 3 hours performed up to five times per week whereby IL-6 levels were increased because of increased muscle activity.[245 246]

2.22.2 Sports & Exercise Training on Palliative Care of Kaposi Sarcoma

An approach can be to improve the quality of life of KS patients by reducing painful accompanying symptoms such as bilateral foot pain due to plantar surface lesions by walking short distances after gait training with the additional use of comfortable plastazote sandals resp. lower extremity lymphedema by isometric exercises for the lower limbs and passive knee flexion with painless range of motion together with the additional use of compressive bandages and garments.[247]

2.23 Hodgkin Lymphoma

Hodgkin Lymphoma represents the cancer with the 23rd highest mortality rate with 25.469 cancer deaths in 2012 worldwide by being the 19th most common and 18th deadliest cancer in 2012 among men resp. the 21st most common and 21st deadliest cancer in 2012 among women with an incidence rate of 38.520 new cases as well as a mortality rate of 15.463 deaths in 2012 among men resp. an incidence rate of 27.430 new cases as well as a mortality rate of 10.006 deaths in 2012 among women.[2] Hodgkin Lymphoma is a type of blood cancer originating from white blood cells called B-lymphocytes being responsible for strengthening everyone's immune system by producing antibodies to prevent infections whereby the only difference in comparison with the Non-Hodgkin lymphoma (NHL) is that the Hodgkin Lymphoma (HL) has got Reed-Steinberg-Cells that can be noticed by light microscope and belong to the afore-mentioned B-lymphocytes. The most important risk factor of HL is the Epstein Barr virus (EBV) causing glandular fever and being related to almost 50% of all HL cases whereby also previous NHL, lowered immunity such as HIV or organ transplant, early exposure to common childhood infections, Hepatitis C, family history or occupational exposure to chemicals may play more or less notable roles.[238] The most common symptom of HL is the occurrence of enlarged lymph nodes in the neck, armpit and groin whereat other symptoms include heavy nocturnal sweating, high body temperatures, unexpected sudden weight loss, abdominal pain, breathlessness due to anemia, infections because of low WBC count or bleeding problems such as frequent nose bleeding, heavy periods and/or tiny bloody spots due to low platelet count.[239]

2.23.1 Sports & Exercise Training on Hodgkin Lymphoma Incidence

A potential correlation was found in a study where 312 cases who had HL and 325 controls aged 19 - 79 years were interviewed about the participation in high-intensity sports and exercise training with the final conclusion that high-intensity sports and exercise training performed at least twice a week for 1 or more months per year led to a reduced risk of HL with the most benefits for those exercising the most for 10 - 12 months per year whereby the results only has reference to women and not men.[240]

2.23.2 Sports & Exercise Training on Palliative Care of Hodgkin Lymphoma

During chemotherapy in HL patients, physical fitness is decreased with simultaneous declines in hemoglobin levels and increases in chronic fatigue whereby a large percentage of those patients reached sports and exercise training guidelines at baseline what could be explained by lower sports and exercise training volumes whereat another study investigated the impact of moderate endurance training interventions of at least 30 min. per day or 150 min. per week on 5 or more days of the week that was reviewed from 13 issue-specific articles with the final outcome that such interventions have got positive effects on cardiorespiratory fitness, fatigue, depression and physical capacity.[241 242]

2.24 Testicular Cancer

Testicular Cancer represents the cancer with the 24th highest mortality rate with 10.351 cancer deaths in 2012 worldwide by being the 18th most common and 20th deadliest cancer in 2012 among men with an incidence rate of 55.266 new cases as well as a mortality rate of 10.351 deaths in 2012 among men.[2] Testicular cancer can be subdivided into seminoma involving germinal tissue and non-seminoma involving all other tissues. The most important risk factor of testicular cancer is cryptorchidism also called undescended testicles representing the absence of one or both testicles from the scrotum whereas other risk factors include abnormal cells in the testicles, fertility problems, family history, maldevelopment of the penis, inguinal hernia being a lump in the groin area, HIV/AIDS, testicular microlithiasis being small clusters of calcium accumulating in the testicles, higher levels of estrogenes as well as lower levels of andro-gens.[256] The single important symptom, which can be diagnosed by self-management, for early detection of testicular cancer is the emergence of lumps or other abnormalities of the testicles combined with a heavy feel-ing in the testicles.[257]

2.24.1 Sports & Exercise Training on Testicular Cancer Incidence

In 2000, a case-control study containing 212 cases and 251 controls aged
20 - 74 years revealed that frequent moderate- to high-intensity physical
activity at young age of at least 20 min. performed more than five times
per week even increases risk of testicular cancer whereby vigorous physical activity of at least 6 hours per week may solely reduce the risk of
non-seminoma.[258] [259] Because of the simple fact that afore-mentioned
hormonal disturbances of female and male sexual hormones also bring
about increased risk of testicular cancer, studies in the recent past
showed that the most common endocrine abnormalities in testicular cancer patients are highly above-average gonadotropin levels including follitropine (FSH) and lutropin (LH) being both responsible for the stimulation of female sexual hormones such as estradiol, as well as below-
average testosterone levels that cannot be significantly modified by typical oncological treatments such as surgery or chemotherapy.[260] [261] A
study involving 362 subjects aged 20 - 40 years from 2002 - 2006 investigated the impact of a 60-week moderate-intensity resp. a 60-week high-
intensity endurance training on the treadmill of 5 weekly sessions of 120
min. at 60% resp. 80% of the maximal oxygen uptake (VO_{2max}) being
previously tested by inclined treadmill test of a starting load of 8 km/h
and 0% incline and 2,5% increases in incline every 2 min. afterwards
until stopping with the final outcome that testosterone and the gonadotropins decrease after the 60 weeks in both types of endurance training
whereby high-intensity endurance training obtained the most significant
decreases while after a succeeding 36-week low-intensity endurance
training on the treadmill of the same volumes and durations at 30% of
the maximal oxygen uptake (VO_{2max}) led to repeated and slightly above-
baseline increases of the afore-noted hormones.[262] In opposition to endurance training, a high-intensity resistance training lasting about 60
min. with 10 maximum repetitions significantly increases testosterone

levels whereby strong declines shortly after resistance training are accompanied by slow progressive increases with significantly higher testosterone and also DHEA levels by restoring steroidogenesis-related
enzymes after a 12-week high-intensity resistance training of 3 weekly
sessions of 3 sets of 10 maximum repetitions per exercise whereat also
gonadotropins almost remains at baseline levels whereby that was only
tested by 22 men aged 18 - 55 years with a single resistance training
session.[263][264]

3 Summary of Findings in Sports & Exercise Training

In this chapter, the afore-noted studies containing specifications in sports and exercise training type, intensity, volume, duration and frequency are subdivided into endurance, resistance and combined endurance and resistance training in tables. This should form an accurate picture of the spread intensities in respect of prospective studies of cancer treatment in form of randomized controlled trials.

3.1 Endurance Training

The different intensities of various studies being illustrated in **Table 2** are to be assigned to one of the three phases of lactate metabolism being separated by the aerobic (TP_1) and anaerobic threshold (TP_2). Lactate representing the salt of the lactic acid is one of the best ways to determine both turn points resp. thresholds due to progressive accumulation during intensive exertion to inhibit the glycolysis to protect the cells from autodigestion by lysosomes. Within Phase I up to the TP_1, lactate arising in the cell plasma solely in the muscle is transported into cells with higher oxidative capacity causing no measurable increase of lactate that enables long to ultra-long lasting, but only light sport activities. Within Phase II from the TP_1 up to the TP_2, lactate is eliminated into other systems to be metabolized owing to too high levels of lactate inside the muscle that cannot be managed by the muscle itself showing an equilibrium between lactate production and lactate elimination forcing earlier stoppage. Within the Phase III from the TP_2 on, lactate is increased exponentially because of a higher lactate production rate compared to the lactate elimination rate merely allowing short, but intensive periods of exertion. Whereby these two turn points (TP_1, TP_2) cannot be merely defined by lactate, but also by heart rate (HR), oxygen uptake (VO_2), carbon dioxide output (VCO_2) or ventilation (VE), but also the percentages of the maximum power output (P_{max}) can be calculated.[265]

Based on three studies containing 62 young healthy male subjects aged 19 - 25 years being subdivided into groups with regular HR response (n=24), indifferent HR response (n=12), linear HR response (n=14) and inverted HR response (n=12) as well as 10 specific trained race-oriented runners (m=9 / f=1) aged 19 - 54 years, 15 male patients with myocardial infarction aged 59,6 years on average, 13 male patients with cardiomyopathy aged 51,9 years on average and 8 male patients with hypertension aged 57,9 years on average, the following values in **Table 1** are calculated for cycling with adaptations in running and arm cycling.[266 265 267]

Table 1: Percent of maximum for heart rate (HR), oxygen uptake (VO_2), power output (P) and blood lactate (La) at the aerobic (TP_1) and anaerobic (TP_2) threshold in cycling, running and arm cycling.

Type	%$HR_{max}TP_1$	%$HR_{max}TP_2$	%$VO_{2max}TP_1$	%$VO_{2max}TP_2$	%$P_{max}TP_1$	%$P_{max}TP_2$	La TP_1	La TP_2
Cycling	68,5%	85,6%	51,7%	75,5%	41%	72%	1,4 mmol/l	3,5 mmol/l
Running	76,8%	92,7%	66,1%	87,2%	53,3%	79,4%	1,38 mmol/l	3,1 mmol/l
Arm Cycling	63,5%	79,3%	43,2%	63,6%	40,3%	70,5%	1,47 mmol/l	3,3 mmol/l

Table 1 shows calculated values being now taken to be able to show, which intensities are preferably applied on the basis of different studies in **Table 2** whereby % of the maximal oxygen uptake at the point of voluntary stopping (VO_{2peak}) is taken as % of the maximal oxygen uptake (VO_{2max}) and % of the heart rate reserve (HR_{res}) being calculated by maximal heart rate minus resting heart rate ranges from 44 – 50% at TP_1 and from 71 – 84,2% at TP_2.[268]

Table 2: Listing of endurance training concerning different types of cancer by intensity, volume, duration, frequency and effects referring to the 3 phases of lactate metabolism

Author	Subjects	Cancer	Intensity	Volume	Duration	Frequency	Effect	P
Al-Jiffri et al. (2013)	Type 2 DM	Liver Cancer	65 – 75% HR_{max}	3 months	30 min.	3 x per week	Lower aspartate and alanine transaminase	I
Crevenna et al. (2003)	HCC	Liver Cancer	60% HR_{max}	6 weeks	20 – 35 min.	2 x per week	HRQOL	I
Na et al. (2000)	Stomach Cancer	Stomach Cancer	60% HR_{max}	2 weeks	30 min.	2 x daily on 5 days per week	Increase of NKCA	I
Liu et al. (2013)	Ovarian Cancer	Ovarian Cancer	60 – 70% HR_{max}	24 weeks	60 min.	4 x per week	Decrease of ET-1	I
Maimoun & Sultan (2009)	Healthy	Multiple Myeloma	50% VO_{2max}	1 x	45 min.	1 x	Decrease of calcium, increase of PTH	I

Büttner et al. (2007)	Healthy	Leukemia	60% VO_{2max}	2 x	39 min.	2 x	Decrease of WBC and lymphocytes	I
Safarinejad et al. (2009)	Healthy	Testicular Cancer	60% VO_{2max}	60 weeks	120 min.	5 x per week	Decrease of FSH and LH	I
Jones et al. (2011)	Lung Cancer	Lung Cancer	60 – 70% P_{max}	14 weeks	15 – 45 min.	3 x per week	Oxidative status	II
Jones (2011)	Lung Cancer	Lung Cancer	50 – 70% HR_{res}	4 – 8 weeks	30 min.	3 – 5 x per week	HRQOL	II
Van Craenenbroeck et al. (2012)	Chronic Heart Failure	Lung Cancer	90% HR_{AT}	6 months	60 min.	3 x per week	Decrease of RDW	II
Kossman et al. (2011)	Premenopausal, high risk women	Breast and Endometrial Cancer	80 – 85% HR_{max}	12 weeks	50 – 100 min.	3 x per week	Decrease of estrogen and progesterone	II
Fealy et al. (2012)	NAFLD	Liver Cancer	80 – 85% HR_{max}	7 days	60 min.	7 x per week	NAFLD, NASH	II
Colombo et al. (2013)	Metabolic syndrome	Colorectal and Ovarian Cancer	50 – 60% HR_{res}	12 weeks	40 – 50 min.	3 x per week	Decrease of IL-8 levels	II
Heitkamp & Jelas (2012)	Healthy	Prostate Cancer	80% VO_{2max}	60 weeks	120 min.	5 x per week	Decrease of testosterone, LH, FSH +increase of SHBG	II
Rundqvist et al. (2013)	Healthy	Prostate Cancer	65% VO_{2max}	1 x	40 min.	1 x	Inhibition of LNCaP cells	II

Büttner et al. (2007)	Healthy	Leukemia	80% VO_{2max}	2 x	39 min.	2 x	Decrease of WBC and lymphocytes	II
Courneya et al. (2012)	Lymphoma	NHL	60% VO_{2peak}	12 weeks	15 – 45 min.	3 x per week	Improved sleep quality	II
Safarinejad et al. (2009)	Healthy	Testicular Cancer	80% VO_{2max}	60 weeks	120 min.	5 x per week	Decrease of FSH and LH	II
Nagashima et al. (2000)	Healthy	Liver Cancer	85% VO_{2peak}	1 x	72 min.	1 x	Higher albumin levels	III
Tjonna et al. (2008)	Metabolic syndrome	Endometrial Cancer	4 x 4 min. at 90% and 70% HR_{max}	16 weeks	40 min.	3 x per week	Better insulin signaling + reduced blood glucose and lipogenesis	I / II
Bartlett et al. (2013)	Healthy	Lung Cancer	6 x 3 min. at 90% + 50% VO_{2max}	1 x	50 min.	1 x	Increase of p53	I / III
Campbell et al. (2012)	Post-menopausal, healthy women	Breast, Ovarian and Endometrial-trial-Cancer	70 – 85% HR_{max}	12 months	45 min.	5 x per week	Decrease of estrone, estradiol, testosterone + androstenedione	I / II?
Milecki et al. (2013)	Breast Cancer	Breast Cancer	65 – 70% HR_{max}	6 weeks	40 min.	5 x per week	Better dyspnea scale, BP, HR +SO_2	I / II?

Bateman et al. (2011)	Metabolic syndrome	Liver Cancer	65 – 80% VO_{2peak}	8 months	40 min.	3 x per week	Metabolic syndrome	I / II?
Mina et al. (2013)	Prostate Cancer	Prostate Cancer	60 – 80% HR_{max}	6 months	60 min.	5 x per week	Adipokine levels and IGF	I / II?
Baumann et al. (2012)	Leukemia	Leukemia	HR limit of 180 - age	17 months	20 – 30 min.	3 x per week	Decrease of incidence rates of pneumonia and fever	n. a.

(I = assignable to Phase I; II = assignable to Phase II; III = assignable to Phase III; I / II = assignable to Phases I and II; I / III = assignable to Phases I and III; I / II? = assignable to Phase I or II; n. a. = not assignable)
(P = Phase of lactate metabolism)

On this basis of the 24 scientific studies being concerned with endurance training with clear settings, only one study could not be assigned to one of the three phases of lactate metabolism. The majority of the remaining 23 studies took place in Phase I and Phase II whereas in Phase III only 1 study completed the whole endurance training volume. In 11 studies, the entire endurance training volume was completed in Phase II whereby in 7 studies, the whole endurance training took place in Phase I. In 1 study, interval training changed between Phase II nearby the TP_2 and Phase I nearby the TP_1 and 1 further study performed an interval training with changes between Phase III and I. In 4 studies, the settings overlapped the TP_1 that are defined as Phase I to Phase II exertion representing inaccurate specifications whereby in 2 afore-mentioned studies, two groups performed two different kinds of endurance training including one in Phase II and one in Phase I with a better outcome for the Phase II group in testicular cancer, but a better result for the Phase I group in leukemia.

Table 3: Summary of all studies in respect of the 3 phases of lactate metabolism by type of endurance training

	I	II	III	I / II	I / III	I / II?	n. a.	
Cycling	1	3	1	-	-	1	1	7
Running	4	7	-	1	1	2	-	15
Arm Cycling or Cycling	1	-	-	-	-	-	-	1
Endurance	1	1	-	-	-	1	-	3
	7	11	1	1	1	4	1	26

(I = assignable to Phase I; II = assignable to Phase II; III = assignable to Phase III; I / II = assignable to Phases I and II; I / III = assignable to Phases I and III; I / II? = assignable to Phase I or II; n. a. = not assignable)

In general, Phase III models in respect of prevention and risk reduction of cancer are hardly ever researched and implemented in humans except for the determination of the quality of life what should be performed in prospective studies because of positive effects by repeatedly transient and short-term systemic acidosis in form of high-intensity exertion affecting the microenvironment of the tumor and concurrently decelerating its progression from a benign to a malignant tumor.[269 270]

On the other hand, high-intensity endurance training above the LTP_2 can be connected with low-intensity endurance training under the LTP_1 to influence the tumor microenvironment by decreasing angiogenesis, the erythrocyte count and the lactate content resp. increasing the level of oxygen and the pH-value to prevent the destruction of healthy tissue as well as tumor proliferation and metastasis as well as by increasing IL-6, IL-8, IL-10, TNF-α, and MCP-1 and thereby inducing modest elevations of inflammatory cytokine/chemokine levels in the blood.[16][271] Low-intensity endurance training under the LTP_1 can furthermore be helpful in increasing the overall survival and decreasing metastases by manipulating cancer metabolism because lactic acidosis and low glucose levels are common in most cancer cells enabling their survival and proliferation whereby raising the pH-value can convert lactic acidosis to lactosis leading to a return to the Warburg effect bringing about glucose deprivation and the die-off resp. killing of cancer cells.[272]

3.2 Resistance Training

The different intensities of variant studies being exemplified in **Table 4** are allocated into one of the three different resistance training intensities called maximal strength including 1 - 5 repetitions at 85 - 100% of the 1 repetition maximum, hypertrophy requiring 6 - 20 repetitions at 60 - 85% of the 1 repetition maximum and strength endurance including more than 20 repetitions at less than 60% of the 1 repetition maximum. The advantages of maximal strength training are improvements of neuromuscular activation, explosive strength and activation of FT-fibers. The benefits of hypertrophy training are increased number of capillaries, enzymatic activity, muscle mass and also maximum strength. Strength endurance is pre-eminently advantageous in developing a higher number of capillaries causing better perfusion as well as better enzymatic activity and muscle endurance.[273]

Table 4: Listing of resistance training concerning different types of cancer by intensity, volume, duration, frequency and effects in regards to the 3 different types of resistance training

Author	Sub-jects	Cancer	Intensity	Volume	Dura-tion	Fre-quency	Effect
Lee et al. (2012)	Obesity	Liver Cancer	8 – 12 RM	3 months	60 min. and 10 exercises of 1 – 2 sets	3 x per week	Insulin sen-sitivity
Ahn et al. (2013)	Colon Cancer	Colo-rectal Cancer	Isometric or 12 RM	12 months	7 exer-cises of 10 sec. or 3 sets	2 x per day	Better bowl motility +shorter hospital stay
Kam-stra et al. (2013)	Head and Neck Cancer	Head and Neck Cancer	6 – 8 RM + 6 – 15 sec. stretching	7 years and 4 months	1 exer-cise of 1 set + stretching	5 x per day	De-crease of trismus
Lonbro et al. (2013)	Head and Neck Cancer	Head and Neck Cancer	8 – 15 RM	12 weeks	7 exer-cises of 2 – 3 sets	2 – 3 x per week	Muscle strength and lean body mass
Galvao et al. (2008)	Prostate Cancer	Prostate Cancer	6 – 12 RM	20 weeks	8 exer-cises of 2 – 4 sets	2 x per week	In-crease of SHBG and DHEA
Tre-nerry et al. (2007)	Healthy	Thyroid Cancer	12 RM	1 x	12 repe-titions one set	1 x	Increase of STAT3
Sato et al. (2014)	Healthy	Testi-cular Cancer	10 RM	12 weeks	2 exer-cises of 3 sets	3 x per week	Increase of testo-sterone and DHEA

Rojas Vega et al. (2010)	Healthy	Kidney and Endo-metrial Cancer	40% of 1RM	1 x	3 repe-titions one set	1 x	Increase of IGF-I levels
Rojas Vega et al. (2010)	Healthy	Kidney and Endo-metrial Cancer	40% and 110% of 1RM	1 x	3 repe-titions one set	1 x	Increase of IGF-I levels

Based on the 8 studies, it has to be said that 7 studies performed their resistance training at the intensity of hypertrophy whereas solely 1 study tested at 40% and 110% of the 1 repetition maximum with the better issue for the 40% of the 1 repetition maximum.

Table 5: Summary of all studies in respect of the 3 different types of resistance training

	Maximum Strength	Hypertrophy	Strength Endurance	
Studies	1	7	1	9

All in all, scientific research including intensities of strength endurance and maximal strength should be performed to obtain information about modes of action referring to cancer resp. concerning hypertrophy train-ing, patients with different types of cancer are supposed to be involved in randomized controlled trials to be able to develop new and helpful re-sistance training programs owing to positive approaches in physiological changes, but not solely positive effects on the quality of life including muscular function and body composition representing the key statement in recent studies.[209]

3.3 Combined Endurance and Resistance Training

The different intensities in **Table 6** are assigned to one of the three aforesaid phases of metabolism respecting endurance training as well as to maximal strength, hypertrophy or strength endurance regarding resistance training.

Table 6: Listing of combined endurance and resistance training concerning different types of cancer by intensity, volume, duration, frequency and effects

Author	Subjects	Cancer	Intensity	Volume	Duration	Fre-quency	Effect
Morano et al. (2013)	Lung Cancer	Lung Cancer	80% P_{max} + 15 RM	4 weeks	10 – 30 min. + 15 repetitions per minute	5 x per week	Improved pre-operative functional capacities
Kelm et al. (2003)	Liver Metastasis	Liver Cancer	130 – 150 bpm (HR) + 15 – 25 RM	13 weeks	2 – 3 x 10 min.+3 sets each exercise	2 x per week	HRQOL
Cheville et al. (2013)	Colorectal Cancer	Colorectal Cancer	Brisk walking + 10 – 15 RM	8 weeks	20 min. + 4 sets each exercise	4 x + 2 x per week	HRQOL
Samuel et al. (2013)	Head and Neck Cancer	Head and Neck Cancer	Brisk walking + 8 – 10 RM	6 weeks	15 – 20 min. + 2 – 3 sets each exercise	5 x per week	HRQOL
Moon-sammy et al. (2013)	Ovarian Cancer	Ovarian Cancer	60 – 70% HR_{max} + 8 – 12 RM	24 weeks	30 – 60 min.	3 – 5 x per week	HRQOL
Bourke et al. (2011)	Prostate Cancer	Prostate Cancer	55 – 85% HR_{max} + maximum repetitions	12 weeks	30 min. + 2 – 4 sets each exercise	5 x per week	HRQOL

Perondi et al. (2012)	Leukemia	Leukemia	70% VO_{2peak} + 6 – 15 RM	12 weeks	60 min.	2 x per week	HRQOL
Cauza et al. (2006)	Type 2 Diabetes	Pancreatic Cancer and NHL	60% VO_{2peak} + 10 – 15 RM	4 months	20 min. + 1 set each 6 exercises	3 x per week	Improved lipid profile of type 2 diabetes mellitus patients
Brooks & Ferro (2012)	Hyper-tension	Kidney Cancer	65% HR_{res} + 8 – 25 RM	12 months	40 min. + 2 sets each 10 exercises	3 x + 2 – 3 x per week	Reducing hyper-tension

On the strength of those 9 studies, the final conclusion is that 3 studies performed Phase I endurance training combined with hypertrophy training, 2 studies mixed together Phase II endurance training and hypertrophy training as well as 1 study each performed Phase II endurance with hypertrophy to strength endurance training, Phase I to Phase II endurance with strength endurance training and Phase III endurance with hypertrophy training whereat 1 further study had to be excluded because of insufficient information concerning endurance training with 130 – 150 heartbeats per minute (bpm) but valid information referring to resistance training by applying hypertrophy training.

Table 7: Summary of all studies in respect of the 3 phases of lactate metabolism and the 3 different types of resistance training

	Phase I + Hypertrophy	Phase II + Hypertrophy	Phase II + Hypertrophy / Strength Endurance	Phase I / II + Strength Endurance	Phase III + Hypertrophy	n. a.	
Studies	3	2	1	1	1	1	9

By virtue of approximate, but not accurate settings mainly concerning endurance training, further studies in form of randomized controlled trials including patients with different types of cancer as mentioned before shall be performed to obtain more information also except the improvement of the quality of life by treating the declining physical capacity of cancer patients that has already been researched and confirmed by combining high-intensity endurance training above LTP_2 with high-intensity resistance training at maximal strength resp. hypertrophy levels.[269]

4 Conclusion

Generally speaking, there are certain and partially significant differences between cancer types due to different severities of verifiable scientific studies that are illustrated in **Table 8** resp. in the above-listed **Tables 2, 4 and 6** in regard to randomized controlled trials emphasizing different effects on different types of cancer with most studies in Phase II endurance training in view of lactate metabolism and in hypertrophy resistance training giving more potential for prospective studies. Breast, liver and prostate cancer have got highly probable evidence in preventing and reducing cancer incidence, progression and mortality because of the most detailed, widespread and directly provable effective sports and exercise training intervention targets regarding sports and exercise training type, frequency, duration and intensity resp. well-established and potential risk factors whereas lung, ovarian, kidney, endometrial and testicular cancer as well as leukemia and multiple myeloma have got probable evidence because of also detailed, but less widespread and directly provable effective sports and exercise training intervention targets. The risks of colorectal, stomach, head and neck, brain and thyroid cancer as well as non-Hodgkin lymphoma and Kaposi sarcoma may be inversely associated with sports and exercise training, but each of them merely has got rudimentarily probable evidence what means that indications of benefits are there, but insufficient detailed and directly provable effective sports and exercise training intervention targets are currently available. Last, but not least, no evidence has been found in cervical, esophageal, pancreatic, bladder, gallbladder and skin cancer as well as Hodgkin lymphoma on the basis of no detailed and directly provable effective sports and exercise training intervention targets.

Table 8: Current state of evidence of clear and comprehensible impacts of sports and exercise training on the 24 most common and deadliest cancer types in women and men worldwide

Cancer Type	Current State of Evidence
Lung Cancer	(3) probable
Liver Cancer	(2) highly probable
Stomach Cancer	(4) rudimentarily probable
Colorectal Cancer	(4) rudimentarily probable
Breast Cancer	(2) highly probable
Esophageal Cancer	(5) none
Head and Neck Cancer	(4) rudimentarily probable
Pancreatic Cancer	(5) none
Prostate Cancer	(2) highly probable
Cervical Cancer	(5) none
Leukemia	(3) probable
Non-Hodgkin Lymphoma	(4) rudimentarily probable
Brain Cancer	(4) rudimentarily probable
Bladder Cancer	(5) none
Ovarian Cancer	(3) probable
Kidney Cancer	(3) probable
Gallbladder Cancer	(5) none
Multiple Myeloma	(3) probable
Endometrial Cancer	(3) probable
Skin Cancer	(5) none
Thyroid Cancer	(4) rudimentarily probable
Kaposi Sarcoma	(4) rudimentarily probable
Hodgkin Lymphoma	(5) none
Testicular Cancer	(3) probable

(1) scientifically proven, (2) highly probable, (3) probable, (4) rudimentarily probable, (5) none

As a consequence, more detailed research in terms of randomized controlled trials including patients with different cancer types has to be performed in the future to make progress within the scope of prevention and risk reduction of cancer.

5 References

1. Ferlay, J., Shin, H.-R., Bray, F., Forman, D., Mathers, C., & Parkin, D. M. (2010). Estimates of worldwide burden of cancer in 2008: GLOBOCAN 2008. *International Journal of Cancer,* 127(12), 2893 – 2917.

2. Ferlay, J., Soerjomataram, I., Dikshit, R., Eser, S., Mathers, C., Rebelo, M., Parkin, D. M., Forman, D., & Bray, F. (2015). Cancer incidence and mortality worldwide: Sources, methods and major patterns in GLOBOCAN 2012. *International Journal of Cancer,* 136(5), E359 – E386.

3. What is cancer. Cancer Research UK. http://www.cancerresearchuk.org/cancer-help/about-cancer/what-is-cancer/cells/what-cancer-is Retrieved January 13, 2014.

4. Hanahan, D., & Weinberg, R. A. (2011). Hallmarks of Cancer: The Next Generation. *Cell,* 144(5), 646 – 674.

5. Wang, P.-Y., Zhuang, J., & Hwang, P. M. (2012). p53: exercise capacity and metabolism. *Current Opinion in Oncology,* 24(1), 76 – 82.

6. Wang, J.-S., Chung, Y., & Chow, S.-E. (2009). Exercise Affects Platelet-Impeded Antitumor Cytotoxicity of Natural Killer Cell. *Medicine & Science in Sports & Exercise,* 41(1), 115 – 122.

7. Gould, D. W., Lahart, I., Carmichael, A. R., Koutedakis, Y., & Metsios, G. S. (2013). Cancer cachexia prevention via physical exercise: molecular mechanisms. *Journal of Cachexia, Sarcopenia and Muscle,* 4(2), 111 – 124.

8. Cancer. National Institutes of Health (NIH). http://report.nih.gov/nihfactsheets/ viewfactsheet.aspx?csid=75, Retrieved January 20, 2014.

9. Jemal, A., Siegel, R., Xu, J., & Ward, E. (2010). Cancer Statistics, 2010. *CA: A Cancer Journal for Clinicians,* 60(5), 277 – 300.

10. Ganapathy-Kanniappan, S., & Geschwind, J.-F. H. (2013). Tumor glycolysis as a target for cancer therapy: progress and prospects. *Molecular Cancer,* 12(152), 1 – 23.

11. Pavlides, S., Whitaker-Menezes, D., Castello-Cros, R., Flomenberg, N., Witkiewicz, A. K., Frank, P. G., Casimiro, M. C., Wang, C., Fortina, P., Addya, S., Pestell, R. G., Martinez-Outschoorn, U. E., Sotgia, F., & Lisanti, M. P. (2009). The reverse Warburg effect: Aerobic glycolysis in cancer associated fibroblasts and the tumor stroma. *Cell Cycle,* 8(23), 3984 – 4001.

12. Danaei, G., Van der Hoorn, S., Lopez, A. D., Murray, C. J. L., & Ezzati, M. (2005). Causes of cancer in the world: comparative risk assessment of nine behavioural and environmental risk factors. *The Lancet*, 366(9499), 1784 – 1793.

13. How activity reduces cancer risk. Cancer Research UK. http://www.cancerresearchuk.org/cancer -info/healthyliving/exerciseandactivity/how_activity_reduces_cancer_risk/, Retrieved January 14, 2014.

14. Tashakkor, A. Y., Moghaddamjou, A., Chen, L., & Cheung, W. Y. (2013). Predicting the risk of cardiovascular comorbidities in adult cancer survivors. *Current Oncology*, 20(5), 360 – 370.

15. Betof, A. S., Dewhirst, M. W., & Jones, L. W. (2013). Effects and potential mechanisms of exercise training on cancer progression: A translational perspective. *Brain, Behaviour, and Immunity*, 30(Suppl.), 75 – 87.

16. Verma, V. K., Singh, V., Singh, M. P., & Singh, S. M. (2009). Effect of physical exercise on tumor growth regulating factors of tumor microenvironment: implications in exercise-dependent tumor growth retardation. *Immunopharmacology and Immunotoxicology*, 31(2), 274 – 282.

17. Ballard-Barbash, R., Friedenreich, C. M., Courneya, K. S., Siddiqi, S. M., McTiernan, A. M., & Alfano, C. M. (2012). Physical Activity, Biomarkers, and Disease Outcomes in Cancer Survivors: A Systematic Review. *Journal of the National Cancer Institute*, 104(11), 815 – 840.

18. Kushi, L. H., Doyle, C., McCullough, M., Rock, C. L., Demark-Wahnefried, W., Bandera, E. V., Gapstur, S., Patel, A. V., Andrews, K., & Gansler, T. (2012). American Cancer Society Guidelines on Nutrition and Physical Activity for Cancer Prevention: Reducing the Risk of Cancer With Healthy Food Choices and Physical Activity. *CA:A Cancer Journal for Clinicians*, 62(1), 30 – 67.

19. Daniels, M. G., Bowman, R. V., Yang, I. A., Govindan, R., & Fong, K. M. (2013). An emerging place for lung cancer genomics in 2013. *Journal of Thoracic Disease*, 5(Suppl. 5), 491 – 497.

20. Gilad, S., Lithwick-Yanai, G., Barshack, I., Benjamin, S., Krivitsky, I., Bocker Edmonston, T., Bibbo, M., Thurm, C., Horowitz, L., Huang, Y., Feinmesser, M., Hou, J. S., St. Cyr, B., Burnstein, I., Gibori, H., Dromi, N., Sanden, M., Kushnir, M., & Aharonov, R. (2012). Classification of the Four Main Types of Lung Cancer Using a MicroRNA-Based Diagnostic Assay. *The Journal of Molecular Diagnostics*, 14(5), 510 – 517.

21. McCarthy, W. J., Meza, R., Jeon, J., & Moolgavkar, S. (2012). Lung cancer in never smokers: Epidemiology and risk prediction models. *Risk Analysis*, 32(Suppl.1), 69 – 84.

22. Kovalchik, S. A., Matteis, S. D., Landi, M. T., Caporaso, N. E., Varadhan, R., Consonni, D., Bergen, A. W., Katki, H. A., & Wacholder, S. (2013). A regression model for risk diffrence estimation in population-based case-control studies clarifies gender differences in lung cancer risk of smokers and never smokers. *BMC Medical Research Methodology,* 13(143), 1 – 8.

23. Beckles, M. A., Spiro, S. G., Colice, G. L., & Rudd, R. M. (2003). Initial Evaluation of the Patient With Lung Cancer: Symptoms, Signs, Laboratory Tests, and Paraneoplastic Syndromes. *Chest,* 123(Suppl. 1), 97 – 104.

24. Molina, J. R., Yang, P., Cassivi, S. D., Schild, S. E., & Adjei, A. A. (2008). Non-Small Cell Lung Cancer: Epidemiology, Risk Factors, Treatment, and Survivorship. *Mayo Clinic Proceedings,* 83(5), 584 – 594.

25. Sui, X., Lee, D.-C., Matthews, C. E., Adams, S. A., Hebert, J. R., Church, T. S., Lee, C.-D., & Blair, S. N. (2010). The Influence of Cardiorespiratory Fitness on Lung Cancer Mortality. *Medicine & Science in Sports & Exercise,* 42(5), 872 – 878.

26. Buffart, L. M., Singh, A. S., van Loon, E. C. P., van Vermeulen, H. I., Brug, J., & Chinapaw, M. J. M. (2014). Physical activity and the risk of developing lung cancer among smokers: A meta-analysis. *Journal of Science and Medicine in Sport,* 17(1), 67 – 71.

27. Lam, T. K., Moore, S. C., Brinton, L. A., Smith, L., Hollenbeck, A. R., Gierach, G. L., & Freedman, N. D. (2013). Anthropometric Measures and Physical Activity and the Risk of Lung Cancer in Never-Smokers: A Prospective Cohort Study. *PLoS ONE,* 8(8), 1 – 8.

28. Rundle, A., Richie, J., Steindorf, K., Peluso, M., Overvad, K., Raaschou-Nielsen, O., Clavel-Chapelon, F., Linseisen, J. P., Boeing, H., Trichopoulou, A., Palli, D., Krogh, V., Tumino, R., Panico, S., Bueno-De-Mesquita, H. B., Peeters, P. H., Lund, E., Gonzalez, C. A., Martinez, C., Dorronsoro, M., Barricarte, A., Tormo, M. J., Quiros, J. R., Agudo, A., Berglund, G., Jarvholm, B., Bingham, S., Key, T. J., Gormally, E., Saracci, R., Kaaks, R., Riboli, E., & Vineis, P. (2010). Physical activity and lung cancer among non-smokers: A pilot molecular epidemiologic study within EPIC. *Biomarkers,* 15(1), 20 – 30.

29. Valavanidis, A., Vlachogianni, T., Fiotakis, K., & Loridas, S. (2013). Pulmonary Oxidative Stress, Inflammation and Cancer: Respirable Particulate Matter, Fibrous Dusts and Ozone as Major Causes of Lung Carcinogenesis through Reactive Oxygen Species Mechanisms. *International Journal of Environmental Research and Public Health,* 10(9), 3886 – 3907.

30. Jones, L. W., Eves, N. D., Spasojevic, I., Wang, F., & Il'yasova, D. (2011). Effects of Aerobic Training on Oxidative Status in Postsurgical Non-Small Cell Lung Cancer Patients. *Lung Cancer,* 72(1), 45 – 51.

31. Sinthupibulyakit, C., Ittarat, W., St. Clair, W. H., & St. Clair, D. K. (2010). p53 protects lung cancer cells against metabolic stress. *International Journal of Oncology,* 37(6), 1575 – 1581.

32. Bartlett, J. D., Louhelainen, J., Iqbal, Z., Cochran, A. J., Gibala, M. J., Gregson, W., Close, G. L., Drust, B., & Morton, J. P. (2013). Reduced carbohydrate availability enhances exercise-induced p53 signaling in human skeletal muscle: implications for mitochondrial biogenesis. *American Journal of Physiology. Regulative, Integrative and Comparative Physiology,* 304(6), 450 – 458.

33. Koma, Y., Onishi, A., Matsuoka, H., Oda, N., Yokota, N., Matsumoto, Y., Koyama, M., Okada, N., Nakashima, N., Masuya, D., Yoshimatsu, H., & Suzuki, Y. (2013). Increased Red Blood Cell Distribution Width Associates with Cancer Stage and Prognosis in Patients with Lung Cancer. *PLoS ONE,* 8(11), 1 – 7.

34. Van Craenenbroeck, E. M., Pelle, A. J., Beckers, P. J., Possemiers, N. M., Ramakers, C., Vrints, C. J., Van Hoof, V., Denollet, J., & Conraads, V. M. (2012). Red cell distribution width as a marker of impaired exercise tolerance in patients with chronic heart failure. *European Journal of Heart Failure,* 14(1), 54 – 60.

35. Morano, M. T., Araujo, A. S., Nascimento, F. B., da Silva, G. F., Mesquita, R., Pinto, J. S., de Moraes Filho, M. O., & Pereira, E. D. (2013). Preoperative pulmonary rehabilitation versus chest physical therapy in patients undergoing lung cancer resection: a pilot randomized controlled trial. *Archives of Physical Medicine & Rehabilitation,* 94(1), 53 – 58.

36. Yilmaz, E., Özalevli, S., Ersöz, H., Yegin, A., Önen, A., & Akkoclu, A. (2013). Comparison of health-related the quality of life and exercise capacity according to stages in patients with non-small cell lung cancer. *Tuberk Toraks,* 61(2), 131 – 139.

37. Jones, L. W. (2011). Physical Activity and Lung Cancer Survivorship. *CAP Lung Cancer Medical Writers' Circle,* 1 – 17.

38. Baojiang, L., Tingting, L., Gang, L., & Li, Z. (2012). Male breast cancer: A retrospective study comparing survival with female breast cancer. *Oncology Letters,* 4(4), 642 – 646.

39. Kang, H. J., Hong, Y. B., Yi, Y. W., Cho, C.-H., Wang, A., & Bae, I. (2013). The correlations between BRCA1 defect and environmental factors in the risk of breast cancer. *The Journal of Toxicological Sciences,* 38(3), 355 – 361.

40. Peel, J. B., Sui, X., Adams, S. A., Hebert, J. R., Hardin, J. W., & Blair, S. N. (2009). A prospective study of cardiorespiratory fitness and breast cancer mortality. *Medicine & Science in Sports & Exercise,* 41(4), 742 – 748.

41. Davies, N. J., Batehup, L., & Thomas, R. (2011). The role of diet and physical activity in breast, colorectal, and prostate cancer survivorship: a review of the literature. *British Journal of Cancer,* 105(Suppl. 1), 52 – 73.

42. Kossman, D. A., Williams, N. I., Domchek, S. M., Kurzer, M. S., Stopfer, J. E., & Schmitz, K. H. (2011). Exercise lowers estrogen and progesterone levels in premenopausal women at high risk of breast cancer. *Journal of Applied Physiology,* 111(6), 1687 – 1693.

43. Williams, P. T. (2013). Breast Cancer Mortality vs. Exercise and Breast Size in Runners and Walkers. *PLoS ONE,* 8(12), 1 – 6.

44. Courneya, K. S., McKenzie, D. C., Mackey, J. R., Gelmon, K., Friedenreich, C. M., Yasui, Y., Reid, R. D., Cook, D., Jespersen, D., Proulx, C., Dolan, L. B., Forbes, C. C., Wooding, E., Trinh, L., & Segal, R. J. (2013). Effects of exercise dose and type during breast cancer chemotherapy: multi-center randomized trial. *Journal of the National Cancer Institute,* 105(23), 1821 – 1832.

45. Smith, A. J., Phipps, W. R., Arikawa, A. Y., O'Dougherty, M., Kaufman, B., Thomas, W., Schmitz, K. H., & Kurzer, M. S. (2011). Effects of Aerobic Exercise on Premenopausal Sex Hormone Levels: Results of the WISER Study, A Randomized Clinical Trial in Healthy, Sedentary, Eumenorrheic Women. *Cancer Epidemiology, Biomarkers & Prevention,* 20(6), 1098 – 1106.

46. Key, T. J., Appleby, P. N., Reeves, G. K., Travis, R. C., Alberg, A. J., Barricarte, A., Berrino, F., Krogh, V., Sieri, S., Brinton, L. A., Dorgan, J. F., Dossus, L., Dowsett, M., Eliassen, A. H., Fortner, R. T., Hankinson, S. E., Helzlsouer, K. J., Hoffman-Bolton, J., Comstock, G. W., Kaaks, R., Kahle, L. L., Muti, P., Overvad, K., Peeters, P. H., Riboli, E., Rinaldi, S., Rollison, D. E., Stanczyk, F. Z., Trichopoulos, D., Tworoger, S. S., & Vineis, P. (2013). Sex hormones and risk of breast cancer in premenopausal women: a collaborative reanalysis of individual participant data from seven prospective studies. *The Lancet Oncology,* 14(10), 1009 – 1019.

47. Tworoger, S. S., Rosner, B. A., Willett, W. C., & Hankinson, S. E. (2011). The combined influence of multiple sex and growth hormones on risk of postmenopausal breast cancer: a nested case-control study. *Breast Cancer Research,* 13(5), 1 – 10.

48. Campbell, K. L., Foster-Schubert, K. E., Alfano, C. M., Wang, C.-C., Wang, C.-Y., Duggan, C. R., Mason, C., Imayama, I., Kong, A., Xiao, L., Bain, C. E., Blackburn, G. L., Stanczyk, F. Z., & McTiernan, A. (2012). Reduced-Calorie Dietary Weight Loss, Exercise, and Sex Hormones in Postmenopausal Women: Randomized Controlled Trail. *Journal of Clinical Oncology,* 30(19), 2314 – 2326.

49. Friedenreich, C. M., Woolcott, C. G., McTiernan, A., Ballard-Barbash, R., Brant, R. F., Stanczyk, F. Z., Terry, T., Boyd, N. F., Yaffe, M. J., Irwin, M. L., Jones, C. A., Yasui, Y., Campbell, K. L., McNeely, M. L., Karvinen, K. H., Wang, Q., & Courneya, K. S. (2010). Alberta Physical Activity and Breast Cancer Prevention Trial: Sex Hormone Changes in a Year-Long Exercise Intervention Among Postmenopausal Women. *Journal of Clinical Oncology,* 28(9), 1458 – 1466.

50. Pijpe, A., Manders, P., Brohet, R. M., Collee, J. M., Verhoef, S., Vasen, H. F. A., Hoogerbrugge, N., van Asperen, C. J., Dommering, C., Ausems, M. G. E. M., Aalfs, C. M., Gomez-Garcia, E. B., HEBON, van't Veer, L. J., van Leeuwen, F. E., & Rookus, M. A. (2010). Physical activity and the risk of breast cancer in BRCA1/2 mutation carriers. *Breast Cancer Research and Treatment,* 120(1), 235 – 244.

51. Kobayashi, L. C., Janssen, I., Richardson, H., Lai, A. S., Spinelli, J. J., & Aronson, K. J. (2013). Moderate-to-vigorous intensity physical activity across the life course and risk of pre- and postmenopausal breast cancer. *Breast Cancer Research and Treatment,* 139(3), 851 – 861.

52. Moghadasi, M., & Siavashpour, S. (2013). The effect of 12 weeks of resistance training on hormones of bone formation in young sedentary women. *European Journal of Applied Physiology,* 113(1), 25 – 32.

53. Wu, Y., Zhang, D, & Kang, S. (2013). Physical activity and risk of breast cancer: a meta-analysis of prospective studies. *Breast Cancer Research and Treatment,* 137(3), 869 – 882.

54. Volaklis, K. A., Halle, M., & Tokmakidis, S. P. (2013). Exercise in the prevention and rehabilitation of breast cancer. *Wiener klinische Wochenschrift,* 125(11-12), 297 – 301.

55. Graf, C., & Wessely, N. (2010). Physical Activity in the Prevention and Therapy of Breast Cancer. *Breast Care,* 5(6), 389 – 394.

56. Herrero, F., San Juan, A. F., Fleck, S. J., Balmer, J., Perez, M., Canete, S., Earnest, C. P., Foster, C., & Lucia, A. (2006). Combined Aerobic and Resistance Training in Breast Cancer Survivors: A Randomized, Controlled Pilot Trial. *International Journal of Sports Medicine,* 27(7), 573 – 580.

57. Milecki, P., Hojan, K., Ozga-Majchrzak, O., & Molinska-Glura, M. (2013). Exercise tolerance in breast cancer patients during radiotherapy after aerobic training. *Contemporary Oncology,* 17(2), 205 – 209.

58. Chuang, C. Z., Martin, L. F., LeGardeur, B. Y., & Lopes, A. (2001). Physical activity, biliary lipids, and gallstones in obese subjects. *American Journal of Gastroenterology,* 96(6), 1860 – 1865.

59. Symptoms of liver cancer. Cancer Research UK. http://www.cancerresearchuk.org/cancer-help/type/liver-cancer/about/symptoms-of-liver-cancer, Retrieved February 15, 2014.

60. Berentzen, T. L., Gamborg, M., Holst, C., Sorensen, T. I, A., & Baker, J. L. (2013). Body mass index in childhood and adult risk of primary liver cancer. *Journal of Hepatology,* In Press, Corrected Proof, Available online 26 September 2013, 1 – 6.

61. Gerber, L., Otgonsuren, M., Mishra, A., Escheik, C., Birerdinc, A., Stepanova, M., & Younossi, Z. M. (2012). Non-alcoholic fatty liver disease (NAFLD) is associated with low level of physical activity: a population-based study. *Alimentary Pharmacology and Therapeutics,* 36(8), 772 – 781.

62. Lee, S., Bacha, F., Hannon, T., Kuk, J. L., Boesch, C., & Arslanian, S. (2012). Effects of Aerobic Versus Resistance Exercise Without Caloric Restriction on Abdominal Fat, Intrahepatic Lipid, and Insullin Sensitivity in Obese Adolescent Boys. *Diabetes,* 61(11), 2787 – 2795.

63. Bateman, L. A., Slentz, C. A., Willis, L. H., Shields, A. T., Piner, L. W., Bales, C. W., Houmard, J. A., & Kraus, W. E. (2011). Comparison of Aerobic Versus Resistance Exercise Training Effects on Metabolic Syndrome (from the Studies of a Targeted Risk Reduction Intervention Through Defined Exercise – STRRIDE-AT/RT). *The American Journal of Cardiology,* 108(6), 838 – 844.

64. Bae, J. C., Suh, S., Park, S. E., Rhee, E. J., Park, C. Y., Oh, K. W., Park, S. W., Kim, S. W., Hur, K. Y., Kim, J. H., Lee, M.-S., Lee, M. K., Kim, K.-W., & Lee, W.-Y. (2012). Regular Exercise Is Associated with a Reduction in the Risk of NAFLD and Decreased Liver Enzymes in Individuals with NAFLD Independent of Obesity in Korean Adults. *PLoS ONE,* 7(10), 1 – 7.

65. Fealy, C. E., Haus, J. M., Solomon, T. P. J., Pagadala, M., Flask, C. A., McCullough, A. J., & Kirwan, J. P. (2012). Short-term exercise reduces markers of hepatocyte apoptosis in nonalcoholic fatty liver disease. *Journal of Applied Physiology,* 113(1), 1 – 6.

66. Duan, X.-Y., Zhang, L., Fan, J.-G., & Qiao, L. (2013). NAFLD leads to liver cancer: Do we have sufficient evidence? *Cancer Letters,* In Press, Corrected Proof, Available online 10 August 2013, 1 – 5.

67. Behrens, G., Matthews, C. E., Moore, S. C., Freedman, N. D., McGlynn, K. A., Everhart, J. E., Hollenbeck, A. R., & Leitzmann, M. F. (2013). The association between frequency of vigorous physical activity and hepatobiliary cancers in the NIH-AARP Diet and Health Study. *European Journal of Epidemiology*, 28(1), 55 – 66.

68. Alzahrani, B., Iseli, T. J., & Hebbard, L. W. (2013). Non-viral causes of liver cancer: Does obesity led inflammation play a role? *Cancer Letters,* In Press, Corrected Proof, Available online 2 September 2013, 1 – 7.

69. Peel, J. B., Sui, X., Matthews, C. E., Adams, S. A., Hebert, J. R., Hardin, J. W., Church, T. S., & Blair, S. N. (2009). Cardiorespiratory fitness and digestive cancer mortality: findings from the Aerobics Center Longitudinal Study (ACLS). *Cancer Epidemiology, Biomarkers & Prevention,* 18(4), 1111 – 1117.

70. Kaibori, M., Ishizaki, M., Matsui, K., Nakatake, R., Yoshiuchi, S., Kimura, Y., & Kwon, A.-H. (2013). Perioperative exercise for chronic liver injury patients with hepatocellular carcinoma undergoing hepatectomy. *The American Journal of Surgery,* 206(2), 202 – 209.

71. Kaibori, M., Ishizaki, M., Matsui, K., Nakatake, R., Sakaguchi, T., Habu, D., Yoshiuchi, S., Kimura, Y., & Kon, A.-H. (2013). Assessment of preoperative exercise capacity in hepatocellular carcinoma patients with chronic liver injury undergoing hepatectomy. *BMC Gastroenterology,* 13(119), 1 – 9.

72. Al-Jiffri, O., Al-Sharif, F. M., Abd El-Kader, S. M., & Ashmewy, E. M. (2013). Weight reduction improves markers of hepatic function and insulin resistance in type-2 diabetes patients with non-alcoholic fatty liver. *African Health Sciences,* 13(3), 667 – 672.

73. Nagashima, K., Cline, G. W., Mack, G. W., Shulman, G. I., & Nadel, E. R. (2000). Intense exercise stimulates albumin synthesis in the upright posture. *Journal of Applied Physiology,* 88(1), 41 – 46.

74. Strüder, H. K., Hollmann, W., Platen, P., Wöstmann, R., Ferrauti, A., & Weber, K. (1997). Effect of exercise intensity on free tryptophan to branched-chain amino acids ratio and plasma prolactin during endurance exercise. *Canadian Journal of Applied Physiology,* 22(3), 280 – 291.

75. Kelm, J., Ahlhelm, F., Weißenbach, P., Schliesing, P., Regitz, T., Deubel, G., & Engel, C. (2003). Physical Training During Intrahepatic Chemotherapy. *Archives of Physical Medicine and Rehabilitation,* 84(5), 687 – 690.

76. Crevenna, R., Schmidinger, M., Kellani, M., Nuhr, M., Nur, H., Zöch, C., Zielinski, C., Fialka-Moser, V., & Quittan, M. (2003). Aerobic Exercise as Additive Palliative Treatment for a Patient with Advanced Hepatocellular Cancer. *Wiener medizinische Wochenschrift*, 153(9-10), 237 – 240.

77. Haggar, F. A., & Boushey, R. P. (2009). Colorectal Cancer Epidemiology: Incidence, Mortality, Survival, and Risk Factors. *Clinics in Colon and Rectal Surgery*, 22(4), 191 – 197.

78. Fung, K. Y. C., Ooi, C. C., Zucker, M. H., Lockett, T., Williams, D. B., Cosgrove, L. J., & Topping, D. L. (2013). Colorectal Carcinogenesis: A Cellular Response to Sustained Risk Environment. *International Journal of Molecular Sciences*, 14(7), 13525 – 13541.

79. Astin, M., Griffin, T., Neal, R. D., Rose, P., & Hamilton, W. (2011). The diagnostic value of symptoms for colorectal cancer in primary care: a systematic review. *The British Journal of General Practice*, 61(586), 231 – 243.

80. Spence, R. R., Heesch, K. C., & Brown, W. J. (2009). A systematic review of the association between physical activity and colorectal cancer risk. *Scandinavian Journal of Medicine & Science in Sports*, 19(6), 764 – 781.

81. Howard, R. A., Freedman, D. M., Park, Y., Hollenbeck, A., Schatzkin, A., & Leitzmann, M. F. (2008). Physical activity, sedentary behaviour, and risk of colon and rectal cancer in the NIH-AARP Diet and Health Study. *Cancer Causes & Control*, 19(9), 939 – 953.

82. Pham, N. M., Mizoue, T., Tanaka, K., Tsuji, I., Tamakoshi, A., Matsuo, K., Ito, H., Wakai, K., Nagata, C., Sasazuki, S., Inoue, M., & Tsugane, S. (2012). Physical Activity and Colorectal Cancer Risk: An Evaluation Based on a Systematic Review of Epidemiologic Evidence Among the Japanese Population. *Japanese Journal of Clinical Oncology*, 42(1), 2 – 13.

83. Boyle, T., Heyworth, J., Bull, F., McKerracher, S., Platell, C., & Fritschi, L. (2011). Timing and intensity of recreational physical activity and the risk of subsite-specific colorectal cancer. *Cancer Causes & Control*, 22(12), 1647 – 1658.

84. Sanchez, N. F., Stierman, B., Saab, S., Mahajan, D., Yeung, H., & Francois, F. (2012). Physical activity reduces risk for colon polyps in a multiethnic colorectal cancer screening population. *BMC Research Notes*, 5(312), 1 – 8.

85. Slattery, M. L., Edwards, S., Curtin, K., Ma, K., Edwards, R., Holubkov, R., & Schaffer, D. (2003). Physical Activity and Colorectal Cancer. *American Journal of Epidemiology*, 158(3), 214 – 224.

86. Doll, D., Keller, L., Maak, M., Boulesteix, A.-L., Siewert, J. R., Holzmann, B., & Janssen, K.-P. (2010). Differential expression of the chemokines GRO-2, GRO-3, and interleukin-8 in colon cancer and their impact on metastatic disease and survival. *International Journal of Colorectal Disease,* 25(5), 573 – 581.

87. Rubie, C., Frick, V. O., Pfeil, S., Wagner, M., Kollmar, O., Kopp, B., Gräber, S., Rau, B. M., & Schilling, M. K. (2007). Correlation of IL-8 with induction, progression and metastatic potential of colorectal cancer. *World Journal of Gastroenterology,* 13(37), 4996 – 5002.

88. Ning, Y., Manegold, P. C., Hong, Y. K., Zhang, W., Pohl, A., Lurje, G., Winder, T., Yang, D., LaBonte, M. J., Wilson, P. M., Ladner, R. D., & Lenz, H.-J. (2011). Interleukin-8 is associated with proliferation, migration, angiogenesis and chemosensitivity in vitro and in vivo in colon cancer cell line models. *International Journal of Cancer,* 128(9), 2038 – 2049.

89. Barton, M. K. (2013). Higher Levels of Physical Activity Significantly Increase Survival in Women With Colorectal Cancer. *CA: A Cancer Journal for Clinicians,* 63(2), 83 – 84.

90. Troseid, M., Lappegard, K. T., Claudi, T., Damas, J. K., Morkrid, L., Brendberg, R., & Mollnes, T. E. (2004). Exercise reduces plasma levels of the chemokines MCP-1 and IL-8 in subjects with the metabolic syndrome. *European Heart Journal,* 25(4), 349 – 355.

91. Colombo, C. M., de Macedo, R. M., Fernandes-Silva, M. M., Caporal, A. M., Stinghen, A. E., Constantini, C. R., Baena, C. P., Guarita-Souza, L. C., & Faria-Neto, J. R. (2013). Short-term effects of moderate intensity physical activity in patients with metabolic syndrome. *Einstein,* 11(3), 324 – 330.

92. Ahn, K.-Y., Hur, H., Kim, D.-H., Min, J., Jeong, D. H., Chu, S. H., Lee, J. L., Ligibel, J. A., Meyerhardt, J. A., Jones, L. W., Jeon, J. Y., & Kim, N. K. (2013). The effects of inpatient exercise therapy on the length of hospital stay in stages I – III colon cancer patients: randomized controlled trial. *International Journal of Colorectal Disease,* 28(5), 643 – 651.

93. Cheville, A. L., Kollasch, J., Vandenberg, J., Shen, T., Grothey, A., Gamble, G., & Basford, J. R. (2013). A Home-Based Exercise Program to Improve Function, Fatigue, and Sleep Quality in Patients With Stage IV Lung and Colorectal Cancer: A Randomized Controlled Trial. *Journal of Pain and Symptom Management,* 45(5), 811 – 821.

94. Lee, Y. Y., & Derakhshan, M. H. (2013). Environmental and Lifestyle Risk Factors of Gastric Cancer. *Archives of Iranian Medicine,* 16(6), 358 – 365.

95. Yoon, J. M., Son, K. Y., Eom, C. S., Durrance, D., & Park, S. M. (2013). Pre-existing diabetes mellitus increases the risk of gastric cancer. *World Journal of Gastroenterology,* 19(6), 936 – 945.

96. Xu, J., Evans, T. R. J., Coon, C., Copley-Merriman, K., & Su, Y. (2013). Measuring patient-reported outcomes in advanced gastric cancer. *e cancer medical science,* 7(351), 1 – 14.

97. Campbell, P. T., Sloan, M., & Kreiger, N. (2007). Physical activity and stomach cancer risk: The influence of intensity and timing during the lifetime. *European Journal of Cancer,* 43(3), 593 – 600.

98. Sjödahl, K., Jia, C., Vatten, L., Nilsen, T., Hveem, K., & Lagergren, J. (2008). Body Mass and Physical Activity and Risk of Gastric Cancer in a Population-Based Cohort Study in Norway. *Cancer Epidemiology, Biomarkers & Prevention,* 17(1), 135 – 140.

99. Kruk, J., & Czerniak, U. (2013). Physical Activity and ist Relation to Cancer Risk: Updating the Evidence. *Asian Pacific Journal of Cancer Prevention,* 14(7), 3993 – 4003.

100. Singh, S., Varayil, J. E., Devanna, S., Murad, M. H., & Iyer, P. G. (2013). Physical Activity Is Associated with Reduced Risk of Gastric Cancer: A Systematic Review and Meta-analysis. *Cancer Prevention Research,* Published OnlineFirst September 18, 2013; doi: 10.1158/1940-6207.CAPR-13-0282.

101. Yun, Y. H., Lim, M. K., Won, Y.-J., Park, S. M., Chang, Y. J., Oh, S. W., & Shin, S. A. (2008). Dietary preference, physical activity, and cancer risk in men: national health insurance corporation study. *BMC Cancer,* 8(366), 1 – 17.

102. Moyes, L. H., McCaffer, C. J., Carter, R. C., Fullarton, G. M., Mackay, C. K., & Forshaw, M. J. (2013). Cardiopulmonary exercise testing as a predictor of complications in oesopagogastric cancer surgery. *Annals of the Royal College of Surgeons of England,* 95(2), 125 – 130.

103. Na, Y.-M., Kim, M.-Y., Kim, Y.-K., Ha, Y.-R., & Yoon, D. S. (2000). Exercise Therapy Effect on Natural Killer Cell Cytotoxic Activity in Stomach Cancer Patients After Curative Surgery. *Archives of Physical Medicine and Rehabilitation,* 81(6), 777 – 779.

104. Choi, J. Y., & Kang, H. S. (2012). Effects of a Home-based Exercise Program for Patients with Stomach Cancer Receiving Oral Chemotherapy after Surgery. *Journal of Korean Academy of Nursing,* 42(1), 95 – 104.

105. Chelimo, C., Wouldes, T. A., Cameron, L. D., & Elwood, J. M. (2013). Risk factors for and prevention of human papillomavirus (HPV), genital warts and cervical cancer. *Journal of Infection,* 66(3), 207 – 217.

106. Kumar, R. V., & Bhasker, S. (2013). Potential opportunities to reduce cervical cancer by addressing risk factors other than HPV. *Journal of Gynecologic Oncology,* 24(4), 295 – 297.

107. Lim, A. W. W., Forbes, L. J. L., Rosenthal, A. N., Raju, K. S., & Ramirez, A.-J. (2013). Measuring the nature and duration of symptoms of cervical cancer in young women: developing an interview-based approach. *BMC Women's Health*, 13(45), 1 – 8.

108. Lee, J. K., So, K. A., Piyathilake, C. J., & Kim, M. K. (2013). Mild Obesity, Physical Activity, Calorie Intake, and the Risks of Cervical Intraepthelial Neoplasia and Cervical Cancer. *PLoS ONE*, 8(6), 1 – 8.

109. Fang, C. Y., Coups, E. J., & Heckman, C. J. (2010). Behavioural correlates of HPV vaccine acceptability in the 2007 Health Information National Trends Survey (HINTS). *Cancer Epidemiology, Biomarkers & Prevention*, 19(2), 319 – 326.

110. Muus, K. J., Baker-Demaray, T. B., Bogart, T. A., Duncan, G. E., Jacobsen, C., Buchwald, D. S., & Henderson, J. A. (2012). Physical activity and cervical cancer testing among American Indian women. *The Journal of Rural Health*, 28(3), 320 – 326.

111. Tokyol, C., Aktepe, O. C., Cevrioglu, A. S., Altindis, M., & Dilek, F. H. (2004). Bacterial vaginosis: comparison of Pap smear and microbiological test results. *Modern Pathology*, 17(7), 857 – 860.

112. Nie, X., Li, M., Lu, B., Zhang, Y., Lan, L., Chen, L., & Lu, J. (2013). Down-Regulating Overexpressed Human Lon in Cervical Cancer Suppresses Cell Proliferation and Bioenergetics. *PLoS ONE*, 8(11), 1 – 9.

113. Radak, Z., Zhao, Z., Koltai, E., Ohno, H., & Atalay, M. (2013). Oxygen Consumption and Usage During Physical Exercise: The Balance Between Oxidative Stress and ROS-Dependent Adaptive Signaling. *Antioxidants & Redox Signaling*, 18(10), 1208 – 1246.

114. Bayot, A., Gareil, M., Chavatte, L., Hamon, M.-P., L'Hermitte-Stead, C., Beaumatin, F., Priault, M., Rustin, P., Lombes, A., Friguet, B., & Bulteau, A.-L. (2013). Effect of Lon protease knockdown on mitochondrial function in HeLa cells. *Biochimie*, In Press, Corrected Proof, Available online 16 December 2013, 1 – 10.

115. Parker, L., McGuckin, T. A., & Leicht, A. S. (2013). Influence of exercise intensity on systemic oxidative stress and antioxidant capacity. *Clinical Physiology and Functional Imaging*, Article first published online: 27 November 2013, doi: 10.1111/cpf.12108.

116. Kamangar, F., Chow, W.-H., Abnet, C., & Dawsey, S. (2009). Environmental Causes of Esophageal Cancer. *Gastroenterology Clinics of North America*, 38(1), 27 – 57.

117. Villaflor, V. M., Allaix, M. E., Minsky, B., Herbella, F. A., & Patti, M. G. (2012). Multidisciplinary approach for patients with esophageal cancer. *World Journal of Gastroenterology*, 18(46), 6737 – 6746.

118. Leitzmann, M. F., Koebnick, C., Freedman, N. D., Park, Y., Ballard-Barbash, R., Hollenbeck, A., Schatzkin, A., & Abnet, C. C. (2009). Physical Activity and Esophageal and Gastric Carcinoma in a Large Prospective Study. *American Journal of Preventive Medicine*, 36(2), 112 – 119.

119. Singh, S., Varayil, J. E., Murad, M. H., & Iyer, P. (2013). Physical Activity Is Associated with Reduced Risk of Esophageal Cancer, Particularly Esophageal Adenocarcinoma: A Systematic Review and Meta-Analysis. *American College of Gastroenterology*, Published OnlineFirst October 14, 2013; http://d2j7fjepcxuj0a.cloudfront.net/wp-content/uploads/2013/10/ACG13_abstract_physical_act_and_esoph_cancer_Singh.pdf.

120. Vigen, C., Bernstein, L., & Wu, A. H. (2006). Occupational physical activity and risk of adenocarcinomas of the esophagus and stomach. *International Journal of Cancer*, 118(4), 1004 – 1009.

121. Kavanagh, M. E., O'Sullivan, K. E., O'Hanlon, C., O'Sullivan, J. N., Lysaght, J., & Reynolds, J. V. (2013). The esophagitis to adenocarcinoma sequence; the role of inflammation. *Cancer Letters*, Published online September 23, 2013, 1 – 8.

122. Vakil, N. (2011). Aerobic exercise and caloric restriction should be the key lifestyle modifications in obese patients with GERD. *Alimentary Pharmacology & Therapeutics*, 34(9), 1133 – 1134.

123. Wasko-Czopnik, D., Jozkow, P., Dunajska, K., Medras, M., & Paradowski, L. (2013). Associations Between the Lower Esophageal Sphincter Function and the Level of Physical Activity. *Advances in Clinical and Experimental Medicine*, 22(2), 185 – 191.

124. Tatematsu, N., Park, M., Tanaka, E., Sakai, Y., & Tsuboyama, T. (2013). Association between Physical Activity and Postoperative Complications after Esophagectomy for Cancer: A Prospective Observational Study. *Asian Pacific Journal of Cancer Prevention*, 14(1), 47 – 51.

125. Argiris, A., Karamouzis, M. V., Raben, D., & Ferris, R. L. (2008). Head and neck cancer. *The Lancet*, 371(9625), 1695 – 1709.

126. Chang, J. S., Lo, H.-I., Wong, T.-Y., Huang, C.-C., Lee, W.-T., Tsai, S.-T., Chen, K.-C., Yen, C.-J., Wu, Y.-H., Hsueh, W.-T., Yang, M.-W., Wu, S.-Y., Chang, K.-Y., Chang, J.-Y., Ou, C.-Y., Wang, Y.-H., Wenig, Y.-L., Yang, H.-C., Wang, F.-T., Lin, C.-L., Huang, J.-S., & Hsiao, J.-R. (2013). Investigating the association between oral hygiene and head and neck cancer. *Oral Oncology*, 49(10), 1010 – 1017.

127. Kubrak, C., Olson, K., Jha, N., Jensen, L., McCargar, L., Seikaly, H., Harris, J., Scrimger, R., Parliament, M., & Baracos, V. E. (2010). Nutrition impact symptoms: key determinants of reduced dietary intake, weight loss, and reduced functional capacity of patients with head and neck cancer before treatment. *Head and Neck,* 32(3), 290 – 300.

128. Leitzmann, M. F., Koebnick, C., Freedman, N. D., Park, Y., Ballard-Barbash, R., Hollenbeck, A., Schatzkin, A., & Abnet, C. C. (2008). Physical Activity and head and neck cancer risk. *Cancer Causes & Control,* 19(10), 1391 – 1399.

129. Duffy, S. A., Teknos, T., Taylor, J. M., Fowler, K. E., Islam, M., Wolf, G. T., McLean, S., Ghanem, T. A., & Terrell, J. E. (2013). Health behaviours predict higher interleukin-6 levels among patients newly diagnosed with head and neck squamous cell carcinoma. *Cancer Epidemiology, Biomarkers & Prevention,* 22(3), 374 – 381.

130. Mikkelsen, U. R., Couppe, C., Karlsen, A., Grosset, J. F., Schjerling, P., Mackey, A. L., Klausen, H. H., Magnusson, S. P., & Kjaer, M. (2013). Life-long endurance exercise in humans: Circulating levels of inflammatory markers and leg muscle size. *Mechanisms of Ageing and Development,* Available online November 25, 2013, 1 – 10.

131. Samuel, S. R., Maiya, G. A., Babu, A. S., & Vidyasagar, M. S. (2013). Effect of exercise training on functional capacity & the quality of life in head & neck cancer patients receiving chemoradiotherapy. *The Indian Journal of Medical Research,* 137(3), 515 – 520.

132. Van der Molen, L., van Rossum, M. A., Burkhead, L. M., Smeele, L. E., Rasch, C. R. N., & Hilgers, F. J. M. (2011). A Randomized Preventive Rehabilitation Trial in Advanced Head and Neck Cancer Patients Treated with Chemoradiotherapy: Feasibility, Compliance, and Short-term Effects. *Dysphagia,* 26(2), 155 – 170.

133. Kamstra, J. I., Roodenburg, J. L. N., Beurskens, C. H. G., Reintsma, H., & Dijkstra, P. U. (2013). TheraBite exercises to treat trismus secondary to head and neck cancer. *Supportive Care in Cancer,* 21(4), 951 – 957.

134. Lonbro, S., Dalgas, U., Primdahl, H., Johansen, J., Nielsen, J. L., Aagaard, P., Hermann, A. P., Overgaard, J., & Overgaard, K. (2013). Progressive resistance training rebuilds lean body mass in head and neck cancer patients after radiotherapy – Results from the randomized DAHANCA 25B trial. *Radiotherapy & Oncology,* 108(2), 314 – 319.

135. Martin, V. R. (2007). Ovarian Cancer: An Overview of Treatment Options. *Clinical Journal of Oncology Nursing,* 11(2), 201 – 207.

136. Gajjar, K., Ogden, G., Mujahid, M. I., & Razvi, K. (2012). Symptoms and Risk Factors of Ovarian Cancer: A Survey in Primary Care. *ISRN Obstetrics and Gynecology*, 2012(2012), 1 – 6.

137. Lee, A. H., Su, D., Pasalich, M., Wong, Y. L., & Binns, C. W. (2013). Habitual physical activity reduces risk of ovarian cancer: A case-control study in southern China. *Preventive Medicine*, 57(Suppl.), 31 – 33.

138. Patel, A. V., Rodriguez, C., Pavluck, A. L., Thun, M. J., & Calle, E. E. (2006). Recreational Physical Activity and Sedentary Behavior in Relation to Ovarian Cancer Risk in a Large Cohort of US Women. *American Journal of Epidemiology*, 163(8), 709 – 716.

139. Mertens-Walker, I., Baxter, R. C., & Marsh, D. J. (2012). Gonadotropin signalling in epithelial ovarian cancer. *Cancer Letters*, 324(2), 152 – 159.

140. Widschwendtner, M., Rosenthal, A. N., Philpott, S., Rizzuto, I., Fraser, L., Hayward, J., Intermaggio, M. P., Edlund, C. K., Ramus, S. J., Gayther, S. A., Dubeau, L., Fourkala, E. O., Zaikin, A., Menon, U., & Jacobs, I. J. (2013). The sex hormone system in carriers of BRCA1/2 mutations: a case-control study. *The Lancet Oncology*, 14(12), 1226 – 1232.

141. Shahzad, M. M. K., Arevalo, J. M., Armaiz-Pena, G. N., Lu, C., Stone, R. L., Moreno-Smith, M., Nishimura, M., Lee, J.-W., Jennings, N. B., Bottsford-Miller, J., Vivas-Mejia, P., Lutgendorf, S. K., Lopez-Berestein, G., Bar-Eli, M., Cole, S. W., & Sood, A. K. (2010). Stress Effects on FosB- and Interleukin-8 (IL-8)-driven Ovarian Cancer Growth and Metastasis. *Journal of Biological Chemistry*, 285(46), 35462 – 35470.

142. Rosano, L., Cianfrocca, R., Masi, S., Spinella, F., Di Castro, V., Biroccio, A., Salvati, E., Nicotra, M. R., & Bagnato, A. (2009). ß-Arrestin links to endothelin A receptor to ß-catenin signaling to induce ovarian cancer cell invasion and metastasis. *Proceedings of the National Academy of Sciences of the United States of America*, 106(8), 2806 – 2811.

143. Liu, Y., Li, J., Zhang, Z., Tang, Y., Chen, Z., & Wang, Z. (2013). Effects of exercise intervention on vascular endothelium functions of patients with impaired glucose tolerance during prediabetes mellitus. *Experimental and Therapeutic Medicine*, 5(6), 1559 – 1565.

144. Moonsammy, S. H., Guglietti, C. L., Mina, D. S., Ferguson, S., Kuk, J. L., Urowitz, S., Wiljer, D., & Ritvo, P. (2013). A pilot study of an exercise & cognitive behavioural therapy intervention for epithelial ovarian cancer patients. *Journal of Ovarian Research*, 6(21), 1 – 9.

145. Von Gruenigen, V. E., Frasure, H. E., Kavanagh, M. B., Lerner, E., Waggoner, S. E., & Courneya, K. S. (2011). Feasibility of a lifestyle intervention for ovarian cancer patients receiving adjuvant chemotherapy. *Gynecologic Oncology*, 122(2), 328 – 333.

146. Giovannucci, E., Liu, Y., Platz, E. A., Stampfer, M. J., & Willett, W. C. (2007). Risk factors
for prostate cancer incidence and progression in the health professionals follow-up study. *International Journal of Cancer*, 121(7), 1571 – 1578.

147. Hamilton, W., & Sharp, D. (2004). Symptomatic diagnosis of prostate cancer in primary care: a
structured review. *British Journal of General Practice*, 54(505), 617 – 621.

148. Heitkamp, H. C., & Jelas, I. (2012). Körperliche Aktivität zur Primärprävention des Prosta-
takarzinoms: Mögliche Mechanismen. *Der Urologe*, 51(4), 527 – 532.

149. Mina, D. S., Connor, M. K., Alibhai, S. M. H., Toren, P., Guglietti, C., Matthew, A. G., Trach-
tenberg, J., & Ritvo, P. (2013). Exercise effects on adipokines and the IGF axis in men with prostate
cancer treated with androgen deprivation: A randomized study. *Canadian Urological Association
Journal*, 7(11-12), 692 – 698.

150. Rundqvist, H., Augsten, M., Strömberg, A., Rullman, E., Mijwel, S., Kharaziha, P., Pana-
retakis, T., Gustafsson, T., & Östman, A. (2013). Effect of Acute Exercise on Prostate Cancer Cell
Growth. *PLoS ONE*, 8(7), 1 – 9.

151. Galvao, D. A., Nosaka, K., Taaffe, D. R., Peake, J., Spry, N., Suzuki, K., Yamaya, K., McGui-
gan, M. R., Kristjanson, L. J., & Newton, R. U. (2008). Endocrine and immune responses to resistance training in prostate cancer patients. *Prostate Cancer and Prostatic Diseases*, 11(2), 160 –
165.

152. Young-McCaughan, S. (2012). Potential for prostate cancer prevention through physical activity. *World Journal of Urology*, 30(2), 167 – 179.

153. Richman, E. L., Kenfield, S. A., Stampfer, M. J., Paciorek, A., Carroll, P. R., & Chan, J. M.
(2011). Physical activity after diagnosis and risk of prostate cancer progression: data from the
Cancer of the Prostate Strategic Urologic Research Endeavor. *Cancer Research*, 71(11), 3889 –
3895.

154. Parsons, J. K. (2013). Prostate Cancer and the Therapeutic Benefits of Structured Exercise.
Journal of Clinical Oncology, Available Online on December 16, 2013, 1 – 2.

155. Kenfield, S. A., Stampfer, M. J., Giovannucci, E., & Chan, J. M. (2011). Physical Activity and Survival After Prostate Cancer Diagnosis in the Health Professionals Follow-Up Study. *Journal of Clinical Oncology,* 29(6), 726 – 732.

156. Bourke, L., Doll, H., Crank, H., Daley, A., Rosario, D., & Saxton, J. M. (2011). Lifestyle Intervention in Men with Advanced Prostate Cancer Receiving Androgen Suppression Therapy: A Feasibility Study. *Cancer Epidemiology, Biomarkers & Prevention,* 20(4), 647 – 657.

157. Belson, M., Kingsley, B., & Holmes, A. (2007). Risk Factors for Acute Leukemia in Children: A Review. *Environmental Health Perspectives,* 115(1), 138 – 145.

158. Wiemels, J. (2012). Perspectives on the Causes of Childhood Leukemia. *Chemico-Biological Interactions,* 196(3), 59 – 67.

159. Karimi, M., Mehrabani, D., Yarmohammadi, H., & Jahromi, F. S. (2008). The prevalence of signs and symptoms of childhood leukemia and lymphoma in Fars Province, Southern Iran. *Cancer Detection and Prevention,* 32(2), 178 – 183.

160. De Gonzalo-Calvo, D., Fernandez-Garcia, B., de Luxan-Delgado, B., Rodriguez-Gonzalez, S., Garcia-Macia, M., Suarez, F. M., Solano, J. J., Rodriguez-Colunga, M. J., & Coto-Montes, A. (2012). Long-term training induces a healthy inflammatory and endocrine emergent biomarker profile in elderly men. *AGE,* 34(3), 761 – 771.

161. Büttner, P., Mosig, S., Lechtermann, A., Funke, H., & Mooren, F. C. (2007). Exercise affects the gene expression profiles of human white blood cells. *Journal of Applied Physiology,* 102(1), 26 – 36.

162. Perondi, M. B., Gualano, B., Artioli, G. G., de Salles Painelli, V., Filho, V. O., Netto, G., Muratt, M., Roschel, H., & de Sa Pinto, A. L. (2012). Effects of a combined aerobic and strength training program in youth patients with acute lymphblastic leukemia. *Journal of Sports Science and Medicine,* 11(3), 387 – 392.

163. Baumann, F. T., Zimmer, P., Finkenberg, K., Hallek, M., Bloch, W., & Elter, T. (2012). Influence of endurance exercise on the risk of pneumonia and fever in leukemia and lymphoma patients undergoing high dose chemotherapy. A pilot study. *Journal of Sports Science and Medicine,* 11(4); 638 – 642.

164. Pandol, S., Gukovskaya, A., Edderkoui, M., Dawson, D., Eibl, G., & Lugea, A. (2012). Epidemiology, risk factors, and the promotion of pancreatic cancer: Role of the stellate cell. *Journal of Gastroenterolgy and Hepatology,* 27(Suppl.2), 127 – 134.

165. Yadav, D., & Lowenfels, A. B. (2013). The Epidemiology of Pancreatitis and Pancreatic Cancer. *Gastroenterology,* 144(6), 1252 – 1261.

166. Halls, B. S., & Ward-Smith, P. (2007). Identifying Early Symptoms of Pancreatic Cancer. *Clinical Journal of Oncology Nursing,* 11(2), 245 – 248.

167. Oberstein, P. E., & Olive, K. P. (2013). Pancreatic cancer: why is it so hard to treat? *Therapeutic Advances in Gastroenterology,* 6(4), 321 – 337.

168. O'Rorke, M. A., Cantwell, M. M., Cardwell, C. R., Mulholland, H. G., & Murray, L. J. (2010). Can physical activity modulate pancreatic cancer risk? A systematic review and meta-analysis. *International Journal of Cancer,* 126(12), 2957 – 2968.

169. Stevens, R. J., Roddam, A. W., & Beral, V. (2007). Pancreatic cancer in type I and young-onset diabetes: systematic review and meta-analysis. *British Journal of Cancer,* 96(3), 507 – 509.

170. Liao, K.-F., Lai, S.-W., Li, C.-I., & Chen, W.-C. (2012). Diabetes mellitus correlates with increased risk of pancreatic cancer: A population-based cohort study in Taiwan. *Journal of Gastroenterology and Hepatology,* 27(4), 709 – 713.

171. Burr, J. F., Shephard, R. J., & Riddell, M. C. (2012). Physical activity in type 1 diabetes mellitus: Assessing risks for physical activity clearance and prescription. *Canadian Family Physician,* 58(5), 533 – 535.

172. Carral, F., Gutierrez, J. V., Ayala, M. D., Garcia, G., & Aguilar, M. (2013). Intense physical activity is associated with better metabolic control in patients with type 1 diabetes. *Diabetes Research and Clinical Practice,* 101(1), 45 – 49.

173. Marcus, R. L., Smith, S., Morrell, G., Addison, O., Dibble, L. E., Wahoff-Stice, D., & LaStayo, P. C. (2008). Comparison of Combined Aerobic and High-Force Eccentric Resistance Exercise With Aerobic Exercise Only for People With Type 2 Diabetes Mellitus. *Physical Therapy,* 88(11), 1345 – 1354.

174. Cauza, E., Hanusch-Enserer, U., Strasser, B., Kostner, K., Dunky, A., & Haber, P. (2006). The metabolic effects of long-term exercise in Type 2 Diabetes patients. *Wiener Medizinische Wochenschrift,* 156(17-18), 515 – 519.

175. Strasser, B. (2013). Physical activity in obesity and metabolic syndrome. *Annals of the New York Academy of Sciences,* 1281, 141 – 159.

176. Touzios, J. G., Krzywda, B., Nakeeb, A., & Pitt, H. A. (2005). Exercise-induced cholangitis and pancreatitis. *HBP*, 7(2), 124 – 128.

177. Letasiova, S., Medvedova, A., Sovcikova, A., Dusinka, M., Volkovova, K., Mosoiu, C., & Bartonova, A. (2012). Bladder cancer, a review oft he environmental risk factors. *Environmental Health*, 11(Suppl.1), 1 – 5.

178. Henning, A., Wehrberger, M., Madersbacher, S., Pycha, A., Martini, T., Comploj, E., Jeschke, K., Tripolt, C., & Rauchenwald, M. (2013). Do differences in clinical symptoms and referral patterns contribute to the gender gap in bladder cancer? *BJU International*, 112(1), 68 – 73.

179. Lin, J., Wang, J., Greisinger, A. J., Grossman, H. B., Forman, M. R., Dinney, C. P., Hawk, E. T., & Wu, X. (2010). Energy Balance, the PI3K-AKT-mTOR Pathway Genes and the Risk of Bladder Cancer. *Cancer Prevention Research*, 3(4), 505 – 517.

180. Koebnick, C., Michaud, D., Moore, S. C., Park, Y., Hollenbeck, A., Ballard-Barbash, R., Schatzkin, A., & Leitzmann, M. F. (2008). Body Mass Index, Physical Activity, and Bladder Cancer in a Large Prospective Study. *Cancer Epidemiology, Biomarkers & Prevention*, 17(5), 1214 – 1221.

181. Burgio, K. L., Newman, D. K., Rosenberg, M. T., & Sampselle, C. (2013). Impact of behaviour and lifestyle on bladder health. *International Journal of Clinical Practice*, 67(6), 495 – 504.

182. Autorino, R., Di Lorenzo, G., Giannarini, G., Cindolo, L., Lima, E., De Sio, M., Lamendola, M. G., & Damiano, R. (2009). Looking at the prostates of patients with bladder cancer: a thoughtful exercise. *BJU International*, 104(2), 160 – 162.

183. Karvinen, K. H., Courneya, K. S., North, S., & Venner, P. (2007). Associations between Exercise and The quality of life in Bladder Cancer Survivors: A Population-Based Study. *Cancer Epidemiology, Biomarkers & Prevention*, 16(5), 984 – 990.

184. Bassig, B. A., Lan, Q., Rothman, N., Zhang, Y., & Zhang, T. (2012). Current Understanding of Lifestyle and Environmental Factors and Risk of Non-Hodgkin Lymphoma: An Epidemiological Update. *Journal of Cancer Epidemiology*, 2012(2012), 1 – 27.

185. Symptoms of non Hodgkin lymphoma. Cancer Research UK. http://www.cancerresearchuk.org/cancer-help/type/non-hodgkins-lymphoma/about/symptoms-of-non-hodgkins-lymphoma, Retrieved January 22, 2014.

186. Pan, S. Y., Mao, Y., & Ugnat, A.-M. (2005). Physical Activity, Obesity, Energy Intake, and the Risk of Non-Hodgkin's Lymphoma: A Population-based Case-Control Study. *American Journal of Epidemiology,* 162(12), 1162 – 1173.

187. Kelly, J. L., Fredericksen, Z. S., Liebow, M., Shanafelt, T. D., Thompson, C. A., Call, T. G., Habermann, T. M., Macon, W. R., Wang, A. H., Slager, S. L., & Cerhan, J. R. (2012). The Association between Early Life and Adult Body Mass Index and Physical Activity with Risk of non-Hodgkin Lymphoma: Impact of Gender. *Annals of Epidemiology,* 22(12), 855 – 862.

188. Lim, U., Gayles, T., Katki, H. A., Stolzenberg-Solomon, R., Weinstein, S. J., Pietinen, P., Taylor, P. R., Virtamo, J., & Albanes, D. (2007). Serum High-Density Lipoprotein Cholesterol and Risk of Non-Hodgkin Lymphoma. *Cancer Research,* 67(11), 5569 – 5574.

189. Bellizzi, K. M., Rowland, J. H., Arora, N. K., Hamilton, A. S., Miller, M. F., & Aziz, N. M. (2009). Physical Activity and The quality of life in Adult Survivors of Non-Hodgkin's Lymphoma. *Journal of Clinical Oncology,* 27(6), 960 – 966.

190. Courneya, K. S., Sellar, C. M., Trinh, L., Forbes, C. C., Stevinson, C., McNeely, M. L., Peddle-McIntyre, C. J., Friedenreich, C. M., & Reiman, T. (2012). A Randomized Trial of Aerobic Exercise and Sleep Quality in Lymphoma Patients Receiving Chemotherapy or No Treatments. *Cancer Epidemiology, Biomarkers & Prevention,* 21(6), 887 – 894.

191. Hoffman, S., Propp, J. M., & McCarthy, B. J. (2006). Temporal trends in incidence of primary brain tumors in the United States, 1985 – 1999. *Neuro-Oncology,* 8(1), 27 – 37.

192. Goodenberger, M. L., & Jenkins, R. B. (2012). Genetics of adult glioma. *Cancer Genetics,* 205(12), 613 – 621.

193. Chandana, S. R., Movva, S., Arora, M., & Singh, T. (2008). Primary Brain Tumors in Adults. *American Family Physician,* 77(10), 1423 – 1430.

194. Moore, S. C., Rajaraman, P., Dubrow, R., Darefsky, A. S., Koebnick, C., Hollenbeck, A., Schatzkin, A., & Leitzmann, M. F. (2009). Height, Body Mass Index, and Physical Activity in Relation to Glioma Risk. *Cancer Research,* 69(21), 8349 – 8355.

195. Komolafe, M. A., Sunmonu, T. A., & Oke, O. (2009). Stroke-like syndrome in a middle aged Nigerian woman with metastatic brain cancer. *Western African Journal of Medicine,* 28(4), 266 – 269.

196. Gallanagh, S., Quinn, T. J., Alexander, J., & Walters, M. R. (2011). Physical Activity in the Prevention and Treatment of Stroke. *ISRN Neurology,* 2011(2011), 1 – 10.

197. Williams, P. T. (2013). Reduced Risk of Brain Cancer Mortality from Walking and Running. *Medicine & Science in Sports & Exercise,* Available Online October 1, 2013.

198. Ruden, E., Reardon, D. A., Coan, A. D., Herndon II, J. E., Hornsby, W. E., West, M., Fels, D. R., Desjardins, A., Vredenburgh, J. J., Waner, E., Friedman, A. H., Friedman, H. S., Peters, K. B., & Jones, L. W. (2011). Exercise Behavior, Functional Capacity, and Survival in Adults With Malignant Recurrent Glioma. *Journal of Clinical Oncology,* 29(21), 2918 – 2923.

199. Bartolo, M., Zucchella, C., Pace, A., Lanzetta, G., Vecchione, C., Bartolo, M., Grillea, G., Serrao, M., Tassorelli, C., Sandrini, G., & Pierelli, F. (2012). Early rehabilitation after surgery improves functional outcome in inpatients with brain tumours. *Journal of Neuro-Oncology,* 107(3), 537 – 544.

200. Chow, W.-H., Dong, L. M., & Devesa, S. S. (2010). Epidemiology and risk factors for kidney cancer. *Nature Reviews Urology,* 7(5), 245 – 257.

201. Cella, D., Yount, S., Brucker, P. S., Du, H., Bukowski, R., Vogelzang, N., & Bro, W. P. (2007). Development and Validation of a Scale to Measure Disease-Related Symptoms of Kidney Cancer. *Value In Health,* 10(4), 285 – 293.

202. Behrens, G., & Leitzmann, M. F. (2013). The association between physical activity and renal cancer: systematic review and meta-analysis. *British Journal of Cancer,* 108(4), 798 – 811.

203. Moore, S. C., Chow, W.-H., Schatzkin, A., Adams, K. F., Park, Y., Ballard-Barbash, R., Hollenbeck, A., & Leitzmann, M. F. (2008). Physical Activity during Adulthood and Adolescence in Relation to Renal Cell Cancer. *American Journal of Epidemiology,* 168(2), 149 – 157.

204. Major, J. M., Pollak, M. N., Snyder, K., Virtamo, J., & Albanes, D. (2010). Insulin-like growth factors and risk of kidney cancer in men. *British Journal of Cancer,* 103(1), 132 – 135.

205. Rojas Vega, S., Knicker, A., Hollmann, W., Bloch, W., & Strüder, H. K. (2010). Effect of resistance exercise on serum levels of growth factors in humans. *Hormone and Metabolic Research,* 42(13), 982 – 986.

206. Wahl, P., Zinner, C., Achtzehn, S., Bloch, W., & Mester, J. (2010). Effect of high- and low-intensity exercise and metabolic acidosis on levels of GH, IGF-I, IGFBP-3 and cortisol. *Growth Hormone & IGF Research,* 20(5), 380 – 385.

207. Williams, P. T. (2014). Reduced Risk of incident kidney cancer from walking and running. *Medicine & Science in Sports & Exercise,* 46(2), 312 – 317.

208. Brooks, J. H. M., & Ferro, A. (2012). The physician's role in prescribing physical activity for the prevention and treatment of essential hypertension. *JRSM Cardiovascular Disease*, 1(4), 1 – 9.

209. Strasser, B., Steindorf, K., Wiskemann, J., & Ulrich, C. M. (2013). Impact of resistance training in cancer survivors: a meta-analysis. *Medicine & Science in Sports & Exercise*, 45(11), 2080 – 2090.

210. Ali, A. T. (2013). Risk factors for endometrial cancer. *Czech Gynaecology*, 78(5), 448 – 459.

211. Pessoa, J. N., Freitas, A. C. L., Guimaraes, R. A., Lima, J., Barroso dos Reis, H. L., & Filho, A. C. (2014). Endometrial Assessment: When is it Necessary? *Journal of Clinical Medicine Research*, 6(1), 21 – 25.

212. Friedenreich, C. M., Cook, L. S., Magliocco, A. M., Duggan, M. A., & Courneya, K. S. (2010). Case-control study of lifetime total physical activity and endometrial cancer risk. *Cancer Causes & Control*, 21(7), 1105 – 1116.

213. Moore, S. C., Gierach, G. L., Schatzkin, A., & Matthews, C. E. (2010). Physical activity, sedentary behaviours, and the prevention of endometrial cancer. *British Journal of Cancer*, 103(7), 933 – 938.

214. Tjonna, A. E., Lee, S. J., Rognmo, O., Stolen, T., Bye, A., Haram, P. M., Loennechen, J. P., Al-Share, Q. Y., Skogvoll, E., Slordahl, S. A., Kemi, O. J., Najjar, S. M., & Wisloff, U. (2008). Aerobic interval training vs. Continuous moderate exercise as a treatment fort he metabolic syndrome – "A Pilot Study". *Circulation*, 118(4), 346 – 354.

215. Ito, K., Utsunomiya, H., Yaegashi, N., & Sasano, H. (2007). Biological Roles of Estrogen and Progesterone in Human Endometrial Carcinoma – New developments in potential endocrine therapy for endometrial cancer. *Endocrine Journal*, 54(5), 667 – 679.

216. Gunter, M. J., Hoover, D. R., Yu, H., Wassertheil-Smoller, S., Manson, J. E., Li, J., Harris, T. G., Rohan, T. E., Xue, X., Ho, G. Y. F., Einstein, M. H., Kaplan, R. C., Burk, R. D., Wylie-Rosett, J., Pollak, M. N., Anderson, G., Howard, B. V., & Strickler, H. D. (2008). A Propsective Evaluation of Insulin and Insulin-likeGrowth Factor-I as Risk Factors for Endometrial Cancer. *Cancer Epidemiology, Biomarkers & Prevention*, 17(4), 921 – 929.

217. Arem, H., Chlebowski, R., Stefanick, M. L., Anderson, G., Wactawski-Wende, J., Sims, S., Gunter, M. J., & Irwin, M. L. (2013). Body mass index, physical activity, and survival after endometrial cancer diagnosis: Results from the Women's Health Initiative. *Gynecologic Oncology*, 128(2), 181 – 186.

218. Randi, G., Franceschi, S., & La Vecchia, C. (2006). Gallbladder cancer worldwide: Geographical distribution and risk factors. *International Journal of Cancer,* 118(7), 1591 – 1602.

219. Andren-Sandberg, A. (2012). Diagnosis and Management of Gallbladder Cancer. *North American Journal of Medical Sciences,* 4(7), 293 – 299.

220. Banim, P. J., Luben, R. N., Wareham, N. J., Sharp, S. J., Khaw, K. T., & Hart, A. R. (2010). Physical activity reduces the risk of symptomatic gallstones: a prospective cohort study. *European Journal of Gastroenterology & Hepatology,* 22(8), 983 – 988.

221. Chuang, S.-C., La Vecchia, C., & Boffetta, P. (2009). Liver cancer: Descriptive epidemiology and risk factors other than HBV and HCV infection. *Cancer Letters,* 286(1), 9 – 14.

222. Koura, D. T., & Langston, A. A. (2013). Inherited predisposition to multiple myeloma. *Therapeutic Advances in Hematology,* 4(4), 291 – 297.

223. Khan, M. M. H., Mori, M., Sakauchi, F., Matsuo, K., Ozasa, K., & Tamakoshi, A. (2006). Risk Factors for Multiple Myeloma: Evidence from the Japan Collaborative Cohort (JACC) Study. *Asian Pacific Journal of Cancer Prevention,* 7(4), 575 – 581.

224. Talamo, G., Farooq, U., Zangari, M., Liao, J., Dolloff, N. G., Loughran, T. P., & Epner, E. (2010). Beyond the CRAB symptoms: a study of presenting clinical manifestations of multiple myeloma. *Clinical Lymphoma, Myeloma & Leukemia,* 10(6), 464 – 468.

225. Birmann, B. M., Giovannucci, E., Rosner, B., Anderson, K. C., & Colditz, G. A. (2007). Body Mass Index, Physical Activity, and Risk of Multiple Myeloma. *Cancer Epidemiology, Biomarkers & Prevention,* 16(7), 1474 – 1478.

226. Maimoun, L., & Sultan, C. (2009). Effect of Physical Activity on Calcium Homeostasis and Calciotropic Hormones: A Review. *Calcified Tissue International,* 85(4), 277 – 286.

227. Amann, K., & Halle, M. (2006). Prävention und Therapie der renalen Insuffizienz: Sport schützt auch die Niere. *MMW – Fortschritte der Medizin,* 148(38), 37 – 38, 40.

228. Mairbäurl, H. (2013). Red blood cells in sports: effects of exercise and training on oxygen supply by red blood cells. *Frontiers in Physiology,* 4(332), 1 – 13.

229. Nikander, R., Sievänen, H., Heinonen, A., Daly, R. M., Uusi-Rasi, K., & Kannus, P. (2010). Targeted exercise against osteoporosis: A systematic review and meta-analysis for opitmising bone strength throughout life. *BMC Medicine,* 8(47), 1 – 16.

230. Coleman, E. A., Coon, S. K., Kennedy, R. L., Lockhart, K. D., Stewart, C. B., Anaissie, E. J., & Barlogie, B. (2008). Effects of Exercise in Combination With Epoetin Alfa During High-Dose Chemotherapy and Autologous Peripheral Blood Stem Cell Transplantation for Multiple Myeloma. *Oncology Nursing Forum,* 35(3), 53 – 61.

231. Bigley, A. B., Rezvani, K., Chew, C., Sekine, T., Pistillo, M., Crucian, B., Bollard, C. M., & Simpson, R. J. (2013). Acute exercise preferentially redeploys NK-cells with a highly-differentiated phenotype and augments cytotoxicity against lymphoma and multiple myeloma target cells. *Brain, Behavior, and Immunity,* Available Online November 5, 2013, 1 – 12.

232. Samarasinghe, V., & Madan, V. (2012). Nonmelanoma Skin Cancer. *Journal of Cutaneous and Aesthetic Surgery,* 5(1), 3 – 10.

233. De Vries, E., Trakatelli, M., Kalabalikis, D., Ferrandiz, L., Ruiz-de-Casas, A., Moreno-Ramirez, D., Sotiriadis, D., Ioannides, D., Aquilina, S., Apap, C., Micallef, R., Scerri, L., Ulrich, M., Pitkänen, S., Saksela, O., Altsitsiadis, E., Hinrichs, B., Magnoni, C., Fiorentini, C., Majewski, S., Ranki, A., Stockfleth, E., & Proby, C. (2012). Known and potential new risk factors for skin cancer in European populations: a multicentre case-control study. *British Journal of Dermatology,* 167(Suppl.2), 1 – 13.

234. Madan, V., Lear, J. T., & Szeimies, R.-M. (2010). Non-melanoma skin cancer. *The Lancet,* 375(9715), 673 – 685.

235. Melanoma symptoms. Cancer Research UK. http://www.cancerresearchuk.org/cancer-help/type/melanoma/about/melanoma-symptoms, Retrieved January 30, 2014.

236. Skin cancer symptoms. Cancer Research UK. http://www.cancerresearchuk.org/cancer-help/type/skin-cancer/about/skin-cancer-symptoms, Retrieved January 31, 2014.

237. Moehrle, M. (2008). Outdoor sports and skin cancer. *Clinics in Dermatology,* 26(1), 12 – 15.

238. Risks and causes of Hodgkin lymphoma. Cancer Research UK. http://www.cancerresearchuk.org/cancer-help/type/hodgkins-lymphoma/about/risks-and-causes-of hodgkins-lymphoma, Retrieved January 31, 2014.

239. Symptoms of Hodgkin lymphoma. Cancer Research UK. http://www.cancerresearchuk.org/cancer-help/type/hodgkins-lymphoma/about/symptoms-of hodg-kins-lymphoma, Retrieved January 31, 2014.

240. Keegan, T. H. M., Glaser, S. L., Clarke, C. A., Dorfman, R. F., Mann, R. B., DiGuiseppe, J. A., Chang, E. T., & Ambinder, R. F. (2006). Body Size, Physical Activity, and Risk of Hodgkin's Lymphoma in Women. *Cancer Epidemiology, Biomarkers & Prevention*, 15(6), 1095 – 1101.

241. Vermaete, N., Wolter, P., Verhoef, G., & Gosselink, R. (2013). Physical activity and physical fitness in lymphoma patients before, during, and after chemotherapy: a prospective longitudinal study. *Annals of Hematology*, Available Online August 21, 2013, 1 – 14.

242. Vermaete, N., Wolter, P., Verhoef, G., & Gosselink, R. (2013). Physical activity, physical fitness and the effect of exercise training interventions in lymphoma patients: a systematic review. *Annals of Hematology*, 92(8), 1007 – 1021.

243. Kaposi Sarcoma. American Cancer Society. http://www.cancer.org/acs/groups/cid/documents/webcontent/003106-pdf.pdf, Retrieved February 1, 2014.

244. De Sanjose, S., Mbisa, G., Perez-Alvarez, S., Benavente, Y., Sukvirach, S., Hieu, N. T., Shin, H.-R., Anh, P. T. H., Thomas, J., Lazcano, E., Matos, E., Herrero, R., Munoz, N., Molano, M., Franceschi, S., & Whitby, D. (2009). Geographic Variation in the Prevalence of Kaposi Sarcoma-Associated Herpesvirus and Risk Factors for Transmission. *The Journal of Infectious Diseases*, 199(10), 1449 – 1456.

245. Sakakibara, S., & Tosato, G. (2011). Viral Interleukin-6: Role in Kaposi's Sarcoma-Associated Herpesvorus-Associated Malignancies. *Journal of Interferon & Cytokine Research*, 31(11), 791 – 801.

246. Fischer, C. P. (2006). Interleukin-6 in acute exercise and training: what is the biological relevance? *Exercise Immunology Review*, 12, 6 – 33.

247. Harris-Love, M., & Shrader, J. A. (2004). Physiotherapy management of patients with HIV-associated Kaposi's sarcoma. *Physiotherapy Research International*, 9(4), 174 – 181.

248. Pellegriti, G., Frasca, F., Regalbuto, C., Squatrito, S., & Vigneri, R. (2013). Worldwide Increasing Incidence of Thyroid Cancer: Update on Epidemiology and Risk Factors. *Journal of Cancer Epidemiology*, 2013, 1 – 10.

249. Thyroid cancer symptoms. Cancer Research UK. http://www.cancerresearchuk.org/cancer-help/type/thyroid-cancer/about/thyroid-cancer-symptoms, Retrieved February 1, 2014.

250. Leitzmann, M. F., Brenner, A., Moore, S. C., Koebnick, C., Park, Y., Hollenbeck, A., Schatz-kin, A., & Ron, E. (2010). Prospective study of body mass index, physical activity, and thyroid cancer. *International Journal of Cancer,* 126(12), 2947 – 2956.

251. Kitahara, C. M., Platz, E. A., Freeman, L. E. B., Black, A., Hsing, A. W., Linet, M. S., Park, Y., Schairer, C., & Berrington de Gonzalez, A. (2012). Physical activity, diabetes, and thyroid cancer risk: a pooled analysis of five prospective studies. *Cancer Causes & Control,* 23(3), 463 – 471.

252. Cash, S. W., Ma, H., Horn-Ross, P. L., Reynolds, P., Canchola, A. J., Sullivan-Halley, J., Beresford, S. A. A., Neuhouser, M. L., Vaughan, T. L., Heagerty, P. J., & Bernstein, L. (2013). Recreational physical activity and risk of papillary thyroid cancer among women in the California Teachers Study. *Cancer Epidemiology,* 37(1), 46 – 53.

253. Couto, J. P., Daly, L., Almeida, A., Knauf, J. A., Fagin, J. A., Sobrinho-Simoes, M., Lima, J., Maximo, V., Soares, P., Lyden, D., & Bromberg, J. F. (2012). STAT3 negatively regulates thyroid tumorigenesis. *Proceedings oft he National Academy of Sciences oft he United States of America,* 109(35), 2361 – 2370.

254. Trenerry, M. K., Carey, K. A., Ward, A. C., & Cameron-Smith, D. (2007). STAT3 signaling is activated in human skeletal muscle following acute resistance training. *Journal of Applied Physiology,* 102(4), 1483 – 1489.

255. Trenerry, M. K., Carey, K. A., Ward, A. C., & Cameron-Smith, D. (2008). Exercise-induced activation of STAT3 signaling is increased with age. *Rejuvenation Research,* 11(4), 717 – 724.

256. Testicular cancer risks and causes. Cancer Research UK. http://www.cancerresearchuk.org/cancer-help/type/testicular-cancer/about/testicular-cancer-risks-and-causes, Retrieved February 3, 2014.

257. Garner, M. J., Turner, M. C., Ghadirian, P., & Krewski, D. (2005). Epidemiology of testicular cancer: an overview. *International Journal of Cancer,* 116(3), 331 – 339.

258. Srivastava, A., & Kreiger, N. (2000). Relation of Physical Activity to Risk of Testicular Cancer. *American Journal of Epidemiology,* 151(1), 78 – 87.

259. Cook, M. B., Zhang, Y., Graubard, B. I., Rubertone, M. V., Erickson, R. L., & McGlynn, K. A. (2008). Risk of testicular germ-cell tumours in relation to childhood physical activity. *British Journal of Cancer,* 98(1), 174 – 178.

260. Wiechno, P., Demkow, T., Kubiak, K., Sadowska, M., & Kaminska, J. (2007). The quality of life and Hormonal Disturbances in Testicular Cancer Survivors in Cisplatin Era. *European Urology*, 52(5), 1448 – 1455.

261. Pühse, G., Secker, A., Kemper, S., Hertle, L., & Kliesch, S. (2011). Testosterone deficiency in testicular germ-cell cancer patients is not influenced by oncological treatment. *International Journal of Andrology*, 34(5 Pt 2), 351 – 357.

262. Safarinejad, M. R., Azma, K., & Kolahi, A. A. (2009). The effects of intensive, long-term treadmill running on reproductive hormones, hypothalamus-pituitary-testis axis, and semen quality: a randomized controlled study. *Journal of Endocrinology*, 200(3), 259 – 271.

263. Tremblay, M. S., Copeland, J. L., & Van Helder, W. (2004). Effect of training status and exercise mode on endogenous steroid hormones in men. *Journal of Applied Physiology*, 96(2), 531 – 539.

264. Sato, K., Iemitsu, M., Matsutani, K., Kurihara, T., Hamaoka, T., & Fujita, S. (2014). Resistance training restores muscle sex steroid hormone steroidogenesis in older men. *The FASEB Journal*, Available Online January 17, 2014, 1 – 7.

265. Kleinrath, N. (2011). *Vergleich unterschiedlicher ergometrischer Belastungsformen bei Läufern* (Unpublished diploma thesis). Medical University of Graz, Graz, Austria.

266. Hofmann, P., von Duvillard, S. P., Seibert, F.-J., Pokan, R., Wonisch, M., Lemura, L. M., & Schwaberger, G. (2001). %HR$_{max}$ target heart is dependent on heart rate performance curve deflection. *Medicine & Science in Sports & Exercise*, 33(10), 1726 – 1731.

267. Hofmann, P., Pokan, R., Wonisch, M., Fruhwald, F. M., Rohrer, A., von Duvillard, S. P., Brandt, D., & Schmid, P. (2001). Die Genauigkeit der %HFmax Trainingsherzfrequenz-Vorgabe ist abhängig vom Verlauf der HF-Leistungskurve. *Journal für Kardiologie*, 8(12), 516.

268. Hofmann, P., & Tschakert, G. (2011). Special Needs to Precribe Exercise Intensiy for Scientific Studies. *Cardiology Research and Practice*, 2011(2011), 1 – 10.

269. Quist, M., Rorth, M., Zacho, M., Andersen, C., Moeller, T., Midtgaard, J., & Adamsen, L. (2006). High-intensity resistance and cardiovascular training improve physical capacity in cancer patients undergoing chemotherapy. *Scandinavian Journal of Medicine & Science in Sports*, 16(5), 349 – 357.

270. Smallbone, K., Maini, P. K., & Gatenby, R. A. (2010). Episodic, transient systemic acidosis delays evolution of the malignant phenotype: Possible mechanism for cancer prevention by increased physical activity. *Biology Direct,* 5(22), 1 – 8.

271. Zwetsloot, K. A., John, C. S., Lawrence, M. M., Battista, R. A., & Shanely, R. A. (2014). High-intensity interval training induces a modest systemic inflammatory response in active, young men. *Journal of Inflammation Research,* 7, 9 – 17.

272. Xie, J., Wu, H., Dai, C., Pan, Q., Ding, Z., Hu, D., Ji, B., Luo, Y., & Hu, X. (2014). Beyond Warburg effect – dual metabolic nature of cancer cells. *Scientific Reports,* 4(4927), 1 – 12.

273. Behrends, J. C., Bischofberger, J., Deutzmann, R., Ehmke, H., Frings, S., Grissmer, S., Hoth, M., Kurtz, A., Leipziger, J., Müller, F., Pedain, C., Rettig, J., Wagner, C., & Wischmeyer, E. (2010). *Physiologie.* Stuttgart: Georg Thieme Verlag KG.

Printed in the United States
By Bookmasters